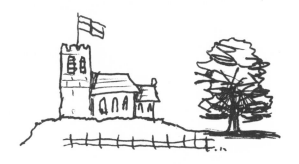

Luella Bartley is a distinguished fashion designer, with over 20 collections to her name. She worked as a journalist for *ES Magazine*, *Dazed & Confused*, *The Face* and was a fashion editor for British *Vogue*. She was awarded an MBE in 2010. Luella currently lives in Cornwall with her partner, fashion photographer David Sims, and their three children.

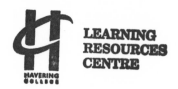
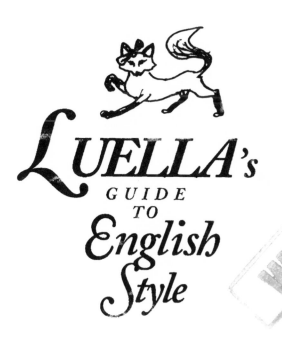

LUELLA's
GUIDE
TO
English
Style

LUELLA BARTLEY

ILLUSTRATIONS BY
ZOE TAYLOR & DANIEL LAIDLER

FOURTH ESTATE · LONDON

FOR STEVIE

First published in Great Britain by
Fourth Estate
An imprint of HarperCollins*Publishers*
77–85 Fulham Palace Road
London W6 8JB
www.4thestate.co.uk

Design by 'OME DESIGN
Printed & bound in China

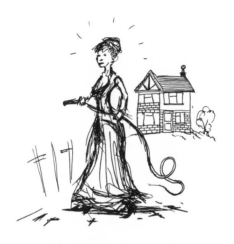

Mary, Mary, quite contrary,
How does your garden grow?
With silver bells and cockle shells
And pretty maids all in a row.

'CONTRARY' BEING THE OPERATIVE WORD

CONTENTS

INTRODUCTION

How to embark on such a veritable romp through the town and countryside of English style? My aim is simply to flag up, carefully and without lasting damage dig up the roots of, and, more importantly, show my unerring appreciation of and devotion to those contrived subtleties and that blatant contrariness that make British women so staggeringly adept in the art of expression through style.

This is not a guide. It might say it is on the front but that's just a cheap trick to lure you in. I just don't believe that it should be that easy. This is more a passionate attempt to infuse the fire back in the belly of Miss England and show how exceptional she naturally is.

There may be some useful info here and there, small insights into the origins of iconic characters, clothes, movements and taste, which one can process and take encouragement from, but in the end the answers to all the questions posed about English style and how to achieve it have to be worked out through a very personal, but ultimately shared, national journey. In a nutshell, this process is the essence of English style – personal discovery and unabashed experimentation with like-minded souls.

In the pages of this book I would simply like to point out that English style is a never-ending labour of love that will result in huge reward (individualism), as long as we don't all get lured to the path of rather undemanding global cooling.

Guiding someone through their style will inevitably kill it. To remain mysterious, it must remain unspoken, but we all need a bit of inspiration along the way.

Not enough? Okay then, the answer is – let's get it over with – a question. It doesn't even matter what that question is as long as it's an interesting question about you. How existential.

It must not be, though, the kind of question that begs the

answer: yes, you are hot. It needs to be a question about who you are and what you want to convey to the world at large about your intellect and your taste. Style is the best way of expressing things about you that are really hard to verbalise. It's what makes clothes for me so fun.

The mix of uptight traditions and unabandoned teenage rebellion that combines to form English style has been an obsession of mine for most of my adult life. The English have this knack of putting together the weirdest combinations of clothing and accessories that somehow – with their warped sense of good, bad and just plain weird taste – inspire the rest of the world. English style at its best is totally natural, fiercely individual and girlishly *contrary*. It can be funny, tough, sexy, clever and perverse, all at the same time. Only in England could frumpy be a turn-on: those public schools have a lot to answer for.

But could I even be so bold as to warn of an impending, perilous doom – duh duh duuuhhhh – for a new generation of Miss Englands, who could easily take for granted the peculiarities of her fine heritage, completely overlooking the eccentric history of her stylish ancestry and her inherent love of the gloriously wrong in favour of convenience style? She may need a kick up the proverbial bottom and a firm hand to turn her from the world of generic, mass, groomed and downright dull fakery that seems to be becoming unnervingly prevalent. Being English is not about being obvious or sexy – it's about being interesting and illogically brilliant. We seem to have lost our appetite for political dissidence through style in recent times. Our most successful style tribes from Punk to Sloanes have been politically opinionated, and perhaps modern Miss England needs to add some more depth to her vintage and irony-heavy character. Has our beloved British bird become a dying breed? I, as a dedicated citizen, feel a duty to protect and conserve her, and her collection of handbags, rock T-shirts, old hacking jackets and found bits and bobs (and their moth holes).

As a designer with more than twenty collections behind me, I've decided to ask the question: what do clothes mean to me? I see my own personal style as a kind of English conservatism, with a grungy, 'bugger it', down-at-heel edge and the occasional sparkly hair accessory. I don't need to prove myself by looking cool any more, although in a typically English manner it took me years of harsh self-scrutiny to get to that point. I've got three kids, three horses, two sheep, a fashion business that just went belly up, a few awards including one from the queen, and thirty-seven years of style ponderings under my belt, a George Sherlock sofa, a very good inherited record collection, a crap car, a vegetable garden full of dead stuff, a dedication from Stevie Nicks, a house in Cornwall where I live with aforementioned animals and children, and a studio in oh-so-trendy Shoreditch. Now ain't life grand? I have a continuing obsession with really old riding boots. I still get a kick from finding the perfect T-shirt – my current favourite is a vintage *Elastica* tour T-shirt – and the perfect pair of perfectly almost faded but still quite blue jeans. I can get away with kidding myself I'm young although I've done the Eighties thing; I was *there* – well, the tail end of rave. I've danced to *WHAM!* in my bedroom while intermittently stopping the tape to write out the lyrics – I was very, very young, you understand – and I've worn ripped jeans, still do, but more out of sheer carelessness than any kind of distressed, *Balmain*-inspired statement. These days I'm more likely to slip on a tan cardi than a pair of PVC leggings, although I'm not about to hang up my sparkly tweed miniskirt just yet, but then that's a post-ironic statement about my approaching middle age.

I'm continually inspired by everything from Punk to debutantes, equestrianism to football casuals, Gothics, pirates, fox hunting, teen angst and all the varying degrees of haircut that come with it, grannies, super heroes, anti-heroes, Cornish witches, geeks, Sloanes, and, of course, The Clash. I have spent the last ten years or so pillaging and adoring British style history while adding a bit of my own to create my own niche brand of English fashion; I know there is plenty more where that came from and plenty more to learn about our wonderful nation. Finally I feel that I have enough experience to embark on this heady journey and get to the nitty gritty of English style and all those who have inspired me along the way. From the sheer rock and rollness of Marianne Faithfull to the epitome of English aristocracy, the Duchess of Devonshire, feeding her chickens in pearls and Wellingtons – both of whom are so thoroughly cool and totally bloody English.

This brings me to another important point, which is that English style doesn't necessarily hail from the notorious square mile of East London that is home to those achingly sublime twenty-somethings whose every waking moment is dedicated to making sure that every centimetre of their attire exists as validation of their superior style. They just spend more time thinking about it, or maybe it just looks that way – you can bet the teenagers in boring middle-class market towns around the country spend as many hours in keen experimentation, it's just the results are less anxious. Some of the finest odes to self-expression and rebellion can be found in provincial towns, as history shows – working-class kids making a desperate bid to shake off the boredom and adversity of being an English adolescent.

Nor is English style determined by age. My personal theory is that British birds tend to get more eccentric, more individual

6

INTRODUCTION

and generally cooler with age. The English granny's wardrobe is a treasure trove of old furs, calf-length tweed skirts, great blouses, pleated high-waisted and belted slacks and, hidden at the back for posterity, the odd Dior gem, a Fifties dress, enough to make Paula Yates drool from the grave. English grannies have inspired the most influential fashion designers, from Marc Jacobs to Karl Lagerfeld – each of whom has a very clever English stylist, Venetia Scott and Amanda Harlech respectively, who undoubtedly have very inspiring grannies. As I write, Mrs Prada has just shown a collection that is an ode to English countrywomen in Wellingtons and belted thick-knit cardies.

Indeed, it is the mature English fillies, from Agatha Christie (and her twinset-clad sleuth Miss Marple) to Vivienne Westwood, the Queen and Maggie Thatcher, who have inspired me in my day job as a fashion designer.

Even without an English granny's wardrobe to pillage, you've got Portobello market – a consistently good place to find the fruits of granny's lavender-scented drawers. 'Oo er missus!' Now, innuendo – and the English approach to sex – is another area that needs to be mined for style inspiration. Think Madame Sin's Streatham bordello (MPs in their underpants), diamante whips at iconic underwear shop Agent Provocateur and Babs Windsor in *Carry On Camping.*

Oh, the French have their chic ladies and their Left Bank intellectualism, the American girl grooms like no other breed, the Japanese take kitsch to a whole new level and the Italians have trash down to a fine art. But the English girl is a multi-faceted dresser with an unrivalled eye for irony and a much more interesting take on everything. Nothing is taboo, nihilism is implanted, mistakes are plentiful and the rules are… there are no rules. Just as long as one adheres to the many unspoken, intricate codes,

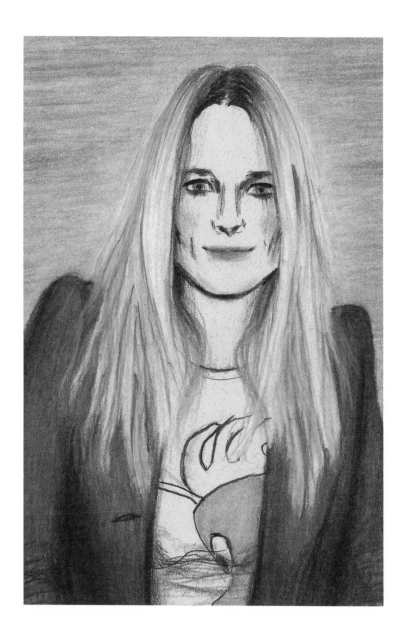

PLATE NO. 1 • LUELLA BARTLEY

ignorance of any one of which makes you deeply, deeply naff (until some cool girl sees the irony in you and then you aren't naff any more, indeed you are a pioneer). Confusing, isn't it? There are more twists than an Agatha Christie novel.

So what makes me such an arbiter? What are my credentials for making such a sweeping fashion statement and daring to turn it into an ode to English style and its heroines?

My bloody baptism took place at Central St Martin's School of Art and Design. I arrived as a fresh-faced, naive, desperately impressionable 18-year-old design student from small-town England. I left Central St Martin's as a shell-shocked, jaded, intimidated and still incredibly naive 20-year-old.

My time at St Martin's consisted of two years of evenings spent in Compton's – Old Compton Street's notoriously wild gay bar – with all my new daring and wild mates (namely the likes of Katie Grand, Giles Deacon and David Kappo), and days either spent avoiding tutorials, drinking endless cups of tea at Café Boheme or rubber-necking in Dave's bar (St Martin's answer to a canteen). Here I would marvel at the competitive eccentrics who catwalked through the canteen to buy their cups of tea and baked potatoes with beans. When I managed to have a one-on-one supervision with a tutor, I suffered the humiliation of having my dress designs ripped apart for being too 'nice'. They didn't fit with the subversive ideas fostered by the college. Back then ugly just seemed ugly, but there was a lot to learn. To this day I have always been suspicious of try-hard haircuts. In fact hair is one of the most telling signs of true English style and the brush its worst enemy – as proven by stalwart bed-head Kate Moss. At points I tried my darndest to be strange but ended up more of a bemused observer than someone with real conceptual tendencies. This was all part of the education though, another step towards the bigger picture.

It was at St Martin's that my deep curiosity about style really set in, but I like to think that my adolescent life wasn't completely devoid of style. My mum spent my formative years floating round our house reading poetry and wearing vintage Chinese dressing gowns and intermittently dyeing and crimping her (and my) hair. That and going to the local college to watch some Punk band complete with fine art make-up that I had watched her apply at the kitchen table with a small mirror and limited light. Good memories. My adolescence was spent in Stratford-upon-Avon and Leamington Spa, sitting in McDonald's after school or getting dangerously drunk (who said teenage binge drinking is a new phenomenon) by night in the park at the top of town (Top Park).Typical English teenage fare.

The weekly under-age disco at Buddies was occasionally inspiring and I vaguely remember Gothic tendencies, such as listening to The Cure. When my coolest friend Beth got a pair of Dr Martens, I felt a huge pang of jealousy. (Beth also went to Ibiza when she was fourteen *and* was the first person at Buddies who knew how to do an acid house dance.) In my later teens I was to spend a year of Saturday nights travelling two and a half hours to get to The Haçienda in Manchester. Yes, I was there, not quite at the beginning, in my mum's Katharine Hamnett jumpsuit or some stretch cotton ensemble, dancing 'til the bitter end to the god that was Mike Pickering. I've been present at my fair share of English youth movements and am unhealthily obsessed with the ones that preceded my years.

But it was at St Martin's that the harsh reality of English fashion really hit me, and where I learned that style and fashion are not the same thing. The realisation that I was never going to live up to the St Martin's idea of cool liberated me, and I jumped at a job shovelling clothes out of the fashion cupboard at the

Evening Standard; post-shoots they had to be returned to their respective designers. Under the satirical wing of the then fashion editor Lowri Turner, I discovered the art of not taking it too seriously, to the point where I had to find Lowri a wig to wear to a fashion show from which she had been banned. This knowledge has stood me in good stead. Self-deprecating humour was what had been missing from my fashion education thus far and is an English trait that can sadly elude those fashion students who take it all FAR TOO SERIOUSLY. Even Punks had the ability to laugh at themselves.

After an apprenticeship of packing clothes, I found myself with a desk on the weekly *ES Magazine* writing a very silly column about fashion called Pony Tales. I should probably confess right now that – like all those other English girls who happily muck out their ponies after school – I've been horse-mad ever since I landed in a saddle aged seven. (But more of the happy marriage between equestrian sports and English fashion later on.) I also wrote a fashion photo casebook inspired by the *Sun*'s agony aunt, 'Dear Deirdre'. This was a pictorial advice column that dealt with issues such as what to do with your unwanted jean turn-ups when they have gone out of fashion (an early Nineties problem sparked off by the jean designs of Helmut Lang which has yet to resurface, although I have sensed murmurings recently).

It was at the *Evening Standard* that my love of the English young fogey look emerged. Some of the male journalistic types, especially those on the diary pages, did a knowing post-Sloane, country-goes-to-town look that included foppish hairdos, lanky physiques, beaten-up cords and Turnbull and Asser shirts perfectly frayed at the collar. Hooray for the silly nonchalance of the toffs – a healthy antidote to the narrow vision of fashion that I had been subjected to at college.

From that cushy number I proceeded with trepidation to the hallowed halls of Vogue House. Never have I thought so much about my outfit in the morning. It soon became evident that my choices were a minor form of scruffy rebellion. I grew to like nothing better than turning up to work in evolving variations of childish contrariness. Everyone at *Vogue* had that experienced fashion look that comes with years of understanding clothes, and what looks good on them personally, matched with a handbag full of discount cards.

At this time my best friend was a girl called Katie Grand who worked on a magazine called *Dazed & Confused* and later *The Face*. She is now a very famous and stylish purveyor of all things cool and fashion. We shared a flat round the corner from Vogue House and used to pride ourselves on making subversive statements like wearing matching fluorescent Gap anoraks (that Seventies childhood staple) with our APC A-line skirts (very Maggie Thatcher) and our ankle-sock-and-Stephane-Kelian stiletto combo (Punk).

Luckily I was hired at *Vogue* for my novelty value and I was therefore allowed my arrogantly enthusiastic mistakes. I was allowed to pursue my, by now obsessive, observations of the English girl. I am still eternally grateful to Alexandra Shulman for humouring me and giving me space in the magazine for my exuberant but naive vision of the modern British girl. While I thought I was being rebellious and testing the boundaries, she simply gave me a knowing smirk.

From there, and spurred on by the drunken camaraderie of Miss Grand – who was striding ahead in making real her personal ambition of launching her own fashion magazine, the hugely influential *Pop* (she is now editor of *Love*) – I decided to start my very own fashion label. My first collection was called Daddy, I Want a Pony, which brings me neatly up to the present day.

Now, as I said, this is not a guide to the perfect faded skinny jean, as important as it still might be to find such a commodity. It's a celebration of all those amazing women from Princess Anne and Vita Sackville-West to Poly Styrene and Kate Bush who have established a very personal but inherently English style. It's not just about Miss England's wardrobe – let that be the name of my typical English girl. It's about how her English eclecticism bleeds effortlessly into her everyday life, giving her a style which goes beyond mere clothes. There's much that must be explored in order to find her essence . . .

So, this is where I'll begin.

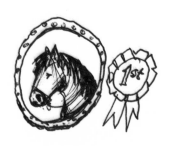

THE SEVEN
STAGES
OF WOMAN

—

The first thing to know about the British bird's relationship with her seven ages is that, in common with morning-after mascara, her style gets better with age. Time is her friend and pure eccentricity only comes with the 'bugger it' attitude, and this builds with getting older. The British bird – Miss England – styles herself with more confidence once she has a bit of history behind her and has made a few mistakes. She looks cooler with a few telling wrinkles. Along with the hairbrush (unless used for backcombing), plastic surgery is an enemy of English style. The lines on her face make it her own; they give her gravitas and sex appeal. It takes a strong character to stay individual under the harsh scrutiny that age brings, but, just as British women are born to take charge, no other female population takes on the challenge of staying creative through apparent adversity. No one embraces their inner outsider like a Miss England.

If a girl manages to keep a devil-may-care attitude towards dressing up through the earlier stages of the seven ages she will have done a very fine thing indeed. There's a tough few years to be had juggling the urge to fit in – wearing the same stilettos as every other hormonal mess out there – and embracing their wanton weirdo geek phase. This is a truly British state of mind and one that every rock star, fashion designer, artist and wannabe creative wants to say they've experienced in their formative years. These early stages happen when raging hormones make monsters out of leggy schoolgirls, rendering them utterly mad and ready to self-destruct. Thus another integral part of an English style education comes into play – rebellion.

Sticking two nail-bitten fingers up at the Establishment, i.e. mum and dad, is how all subcultures are born. Even if she doesn't have the advantage of a working-class background, she can observe the feast of working-class street uniforms at their vivid best in her local city, town or village – and begin to see something for herself in them. From contrariness to full-on anarchy, Miss England manifests varying degrees of rebellion – not just during her pink-fringed Punk-girl revolt at 15, but throughout her seven ages. The arrogance and self-consciousness of her teens – and the designer obsessions of her twenties – are thankfully left behind with the onset of her thirties, which give her a new-found confidence, and in middle age, dare we say it, there's the freedom of maturity.

Growing up is a liberating experience for the English girl – as the years pass, the experimental building blocks of earlier decades start to fit together more easily and her very own, personal sense of style properly forms. What makes British style so unique is the combination of heritage, aristocratic traditions and working-class rebellion – all of which a Miss England can mix and refine to her heart's content, before settling down, later, on the combination which is really her. This, of course, is why an English girl should always look to her older kin for inspiration.

If, however, she doesn't feel that her natural lineage reflects her true, stylish self, then she is within her style rights to look for some new inspiration – think a little out of the box and become the love child of Prince Charles and Poly Styrene. Learning from those who have gone before, British style heroines, or birds as I call them, is the equivalent of sitting at the feet of the village wise woman. It's obvious where Kate Moss's fantasy parentage comes from: Keith Richards and Anita Pallenberg.

I was, to my lasting regret, denied a school uniform. I had nothing to rebel against. My genius of a headmaster made one decree and that was to disallow any forms of tribalism (this clever but eccentric man was also known to sleep under his desk and pick people up by their feet in assembly and tickle them if they were talking). We could wear what we wanted as long as it was not deemed tribal, but this meant no Dr Martens, no gold hoops, no hair dye, no black lipstick. And while this simple disabling of teenage identity made any form of style prejudice or bullying impossible, to this day I believe this headmaster's cruel law was the sole reason for the tardiness of my personal style development. Those with nous, however, could challenge themselves to make up secret style affiliations, ones that would go unmonitored by the untrained eye as we ambled around the parade in Leamington Spa mid-afternoon – truancy was a much lesser crime, you see.

I was pretty lucky with my parentage. A well-matched marriage of a hippy mum who floated around the house in vintage Chinese dressing gowns listening to Fleetwood Mac, and a horsey dude with flannel shirts to die for. Then there's my granny, whose ingenious, high-waisted slacks, pleated at the front, in hindsight were very progressive. I, for one, am saving all my most chic and experimental moments for the final stage of my seven ages. I have outfits pencilled in. I dream of blue sparkly eye shadow and bleeding red lipstick to be worn with my unashamedly tweedy tweeds and comfortable shoes. Oh, I can't wait; in fact, such frumpy treats are already seeping into my wardrobe, thinly veiled as ironic statements. Only when you've got that really wrinkled, lived-in look can you start experimenting with make-up and relive your teenage years of hanging out at the beauty counter at Miss Selfridge, and leaving with a face full of silver and gold.

I say, embrace your eccentricity. You're a British bird, after all.

STAGE ONE: CHILDHOOD — Our heroine is never as free as she is in childhood. How fondly and nostalgically she looks back at her childhood outfits. As a kid it's all about fantasy. One day she's a sparkly tutu'd forest fairy with mum's high-heeled, red patent slingbacks and Ziggy Stardust face paint, the next she's a Power Ranger, teamed with acres of pearls and her dad's trilby. Yes, it might sound a little hackneyed and a little too Hoxton eccentric, but that's only because as adults we are burdened with self-consciousness and rules (no diamonds before lunch, never wear blue and black), rules that we spend the next fifty years trying to shake.

When she's five, Miss England is free to walk down the street in a medley of cute spots, Punk stripes, Glam Rock stars, Deely Boppers, ribbons and fake fur, the like of which Strawberry Switchblade would be proud. And let's face it, *The Beano* is a more original source of style inspiration than any of the more girly literature aimed at young girls. Just think of Minnie the Minx or the Bash Street Kids, for God's sake. We are very lucky as a nation to have such subversive style icons fed to us at such an early stage in our lives. Cinderella, eat your heart out.

Naivety is a little girl's best friend. It means she can be completely free in her decision to base herself on a Tweenie and paint her face blue and her arms in red stripes ''cos it's cool'. Two plus two always equals five – and not because she hasn't perfected the art of addition, although an anti-intellectual position does help at this stage (the imagination must be allowed to run RIOT). Rather, it's about ignoring the idea that everything must be correct and proper. Toddlers naturally disregard the misconceptions that creep up in adulthood – when creativity becomes stunted by rational thinking, conformity and FEAR.

The equations involved in stage one dressing are important

ones. Nothing must add up. If you're really lucky the chaos theory will stay with you for life; you will be experimental and stylish and live happily ever after. British birds are purveyors of the highest standards of eccentricity in the world, and it all starts, beautifully and unknowingly, right here, right now.

Two is the turning point. Yes, by the age of two the English girl has found minor rebellion; her natural tendencies towards subversion are fast forming. Clothes are her first way of wielding control and making a statement – apart from screaming, of course, but where's the creativity in that? No matter how much money an uptight mother might spend in poncey French children's wear shops, Little Miss E will not be told to wear a smocked dress and navy tights if she doesn't want to. She is completely certain of her likes and dislikes and is happy to wear the beautiful, old-fashioned, velvet-collared thing as long as she's allowed her chavvy flashing white-and-pink trainers and her Minnie Mouse ear hat. This is not a compromise, you understand – pre-school style is anything but.

The early development of her innate contrariness tells little Miss E to take a classic and turn it on its head; team it with an ironic statement piece, rip it up, wear her brother's M&S vest *on top*. Somehow it comes completely naturally to an English toddler. 'Ooohh so cute,' is the only critique she's going to get at this stage, which is, frankly, irritating to an angry young toddler with anarchy on her mind. Oh, and at this stage gender is not an issue. Boys are just as appreciative of dresses and nail varnish – a Punk state of mind that segues naturally into the Kurt-Cobain-is-my-god teenage years.

Not to be overlooked is the fact that little girls look great in clothes. Not for them the tricky problems of what does and does not look flattering. And this is where the other vital aspect of pre-school dressing is so important. Proportion. Never does a shift dress look better than on a three-year-old. In later years her legs get longer, lumps and bumps appear and ruin that perfect A-line silhouette. Saying that, though, age has never stopped grown women from taking inspiration from their little style sisters. No one has done it better than the eminently stylish Paula Yates with her pretty pink fairy dresses. Barbara Cartland obviously reverted to her childhood tendencies in old age, wearing her make-up like an overzealous three-year-old and taking tulle to a whole new level. And as Miss Yates and Dame Cartland both illustrated so splendidly, the ultimate way to pre-school-style Utopia is through the not-so-subtle art of accessorising.

Accessories are a key part of this stage where more is most definitely more and a pared-down aesthetic is entirely overlooked. Only a three-year-old knows the power of a strategically placed hair clip.

But the most important lesson we can learn from our little sisters is their ability to show off. Okay, so showing off is a vital part of growing up – posing at the bus stop, standing in line outside clubs – but the swagger and instinct of young girls is natural. Thus the first blissful, unselfconscious stage is over and gone before she even knows what she's got.

STAGE TWO: SCHOOL DAZE — Teenage kicks are a pivotal moment in the English girl's journey of discovery. This is when self-consciousness begins and Miss England's inspiration turns from velour and love heart glitter tights to something more sinister, complex and multi-layered (we're talking T-shirts, not tulle).

The teenage years can be cruel, which is, of course, the point.

How else is she going to push those creative boundaries? Blasting through the pain barrier, in this case, schoolgirl sniggers and taunts, is what it takes to reach a higher state of style consciousness and that contrary, outcast attitude. The lot of the public schoolboy – sadistic masters, flogging and fagging – is nothing in comparison with the ordeal suffered by any girl. Public schoolboys just have better blazers – and better hair.

The key to this stage is humiliation and insecurity, which gives you a big clue as to how Miss E reaches the highest echelons of eccentricity and style. It's all down to the years of hardship.

There are advantages to being a teenager. Crazy charity shop outfits, ripped tights and Dr Martens – they all sit infinitely better on a gangly, fifteen-year-old. Mistakes must be made. In fact, mistakes are very important for the English girl and many are made during these difficult teenage years; some are inspired, some are just plain wrong (which she will soon understand to be a gift, the key to an experimental rite of passage). Both are crucial to an experimental English style education. Self-expression through a hairstyle becomes the most important thing life can offer. Bad haircuts, getting her best mate Julie to cut it *drunk*, modelling for Vidal are an essential part of a girl's evolution. While, at the time, it might feel like social suicide to be seen stalking the school corridor/catwalk in the wrong tights, or Dr Martens that aren't the real deal (Shellys as opposed to Camden Market), the lessons learned enable her to reach the next stage. The scars stay with her and provide her with the necessary character to progress (they do heal with time) and must be accepted as part of the process.

School provides the environment in which Miss E learns about the subtle laws of subversion; here she acquires the secret language in which to converse with others who share the same aesthetic, and usually political and cultural values. School is the great British institution of seditious customisation. Once upon a time Mods wore Fred Perry shirts and loafers to school, Punks added safety pins to their army surplus bags while Skinheads sported budgie cuts and flight jackets over their blazers. Eighties school-yard rebellion took the humble grey ensemble to new historic heights, giving it humour, irony and a clever twist on convention that is sadly missing from those schools today where uniform has been abandoned. This is a thoroughly horrific crime against English style – what is the English school system without a blazer? With no boundaries comes too much choice, which is dangerous and confusing. Teenagers need directives. Who can forget those style-affirming, no, life-affirming episodes of *Grange Hill* that inspired a generation (with or without Jarvis Cocker as an intermediary providing translation to those who missed the glory years) to consider the implications that the width and length of our ties might have on our future friendships and popularity ratings? School uniform serves as a rite of passage that no English girl should miss out on.

FAVOURITE CUSTOMISATIONS OF SCHOOL UNIFORMS

1) THE PENCIL SKIRT — Taking in your straight standard-issue skirt and turning it into something Maggie Gyllenhaal in *Secretary* would find uncomfortable. Your skirt should leave you approximately an inch of movement for walking.

2) SHORTENING YOUR SKIRT — The kind of skirt that prompts the male workforce of Tesco to down tools when you go

shopping with your mum after school (honest, I watched it happen only yesterday). The question is whether your mum does it with a neat hem or do you simply roll up your waistband the cool way?

3) TIES — Short and fat, long and skinny, tiny knots, huge knots, wearing them as a belt, pulling the threads out – all with meanings indecipherable to the untrained eye.

4) SOCKS — Over the knee, scrunched down, rolled down – amazing the variation you can get from a pair of socks.

5) THE BIRO — Essential for customising your bag, shirt, blazer, and most importantly the back of your hand, usually consisting of existentialist statements such as 'PJ 4 Nicki'.

6) BODY DECORATION — Hand doodling can be more intricate than Indian henna. Tippex nail varnish is surprisingly effective for the cadaverous (dead) look. Ear piercing with compass (in dinner hall) not recommended.

7) PIN BADGES — Wearing your heroes, your manifestos, and therefore your cool credentials on your blazer is all-important.

8) SPORTSWEAR — Netball kit. We all subconsciously know the power of this one.

9) JUMPERS — Shrinking your sweater in a good old-fashioned boil wash is the ultimate in uniform sedition. Thumbholes for when you stretch them over your hands are still best for silent angst.

While it is tempting, here, to philosophise upon the meaning of 'cool', to trace its origins back to the birth of youth cultures in the Sixties, suffice it to say that being a teenager is really about belonging to a tribe. The choice of which tribe within the greater tribe, and there are many (of which more later), is influenced by a million (conflicting) definitions of cool. Idiosyncrasies can be as subtle as the number of holes in her ear or the musings on her maths exercise book, but self-expression plays underdog to being a part of the tribe. Once Miss E has found her crowd then everyone else in the world is deeply uncool and, to be brutally honest, beneath her.

But how, without resort to prior knowledge or cautionary tales (unless her mum's still a Goth, which would be unfortunate), does our heroine choose her tribe? It comes at a particularly unstable time; a time of over-emotion mixed with tyrannical rage and painful insecurity, commonly known as puberty and tempered only by listening to existential, misfit pop lyrics – and wearing skinny jeans. Even without the invasion of alien hormones, the incredulity at her body (are these *my* boobs?), who wouldn't be cross when confronted with the kind of cruel attire that she is forced to wear, namely her drab, counter-instinctual, school uniform. Take the worst fabric and cut, put them on a confused girl and make her wear the same combination of grey and burgundy for five days a week and see what happens. This experience will, of course, prove to play a profound role in forming her fashion future by giving her that first, crucial battle with conformity and the Establishment. Out of the polyester cocoon emerges the multi-coloured butterfly.

Lost in her teenage fog, Miss E not only has her iPod permanently attached to her ears, but, avoiding anything labelled 'A Good Teen Read', she makes the natural transition from wanting to be Darrell Rivers in Enid Blyton's Cornish boarding school series *Malory Towers* (the romance of navy tunics and midnight feasts) to empathising with *Carrie* (revenge, powers of darkness) and trying to get her long-suffering mum to part with her hard-earned cash to help her achieve an image of horror. The most frustrating part of forming your look as a teenager is that your mum ultimately has the final say because she still buys all your clothes.

It's a nightmare trying to be like the cool girl (and there will always be a cool girl – mine was Beth Partridge, her dad brought her to school in a beaten-up Rolls) who goes through life with an ease that is, frankly, unfair. Miss E may be discovering her individuality but this is in context of being part of the group, dressing the same as her best friend. It is a lonely business. Tears are as inevitable as slamming doors, braces and nicotine. Miss E's chief concerns are hanging on to her virginity, or desperately trying to leave it behind her, and avoiding an eating disorder. No one understands her predicament, least of all her dear mother, who could well be wearing vintage Dior, but in the eyes of our contrary little Miss E just looks embarrassing.

'You just don't understand,' complains our heroine pitifully and in the painfully nostalgic wail that has become a national cliché in the form of Harry Enfield's genius creation – Kevin the teenager.

By the way, there is no irony in the teenage tribe; that comes later. This is the most sincere form of lifestyle – and dressing – she will ever know. And the only time in her life when patchouli oil actually smells good.

STAGE THREE: RECESSIONISTA — They say that England is at its most creative in recession, another example of how this wonderfully perverse nation thrives on old-fashioned toil and hardship. The third stage of the English girl's style evolution (the charity shop years) is the equivalent of going through a personal recession. Miss England is either at university or art college, depending on her taste in men and academia, or on an indeterminate gap year discovering stuff, or on the first and shockingly paid, if paid at all, rung of her chosen career ladder. There is very little ready cash in the pot for fashion purchases, unless, of course, she's an inheritance-laden bohemian who couldn't care less for any lifestyle protocol, or a new-monied princess, or the girlfriend of a footballer (the latter two being worryingly prevalent in our new cash-without-class society).

Money-is-no-object thinking comes at a price. Too much cash means zero creativity and none of the groundwork or lineage needed to figure out what makes a good status purchase. You're not going to find your true self poncing around Harvey Nichols until you've done your apprenticeship in the markets, high street, charity shops and jumble sales, experimenting, altering, and making proper, individual, out-there choices – and mistakes.

Scouring the racks of Cancer Research is as important to an English girl's further education as A levels and degrees. It constitutes the foundation course for dressing. In the same way that she's chucking paint at a canvas and collaging bits out of magazines in the name of art, so is she throwing together Eighties belts, Fifties sandals and ethnic earrings in the name of style. Invention is the key to self-invention. The English girl will spend hours, days, weeks searching through piles of unwanted crap on Golborne Road and Brick Lane. The Red Cross and Oxfam shops of London's smarter areas (Kensington and Chelsea) and more affluent suburbs (Wimbledon, Kingston) might turn up a piece of eccentric old lady couture for £2. Field trips must be organised to the far-flung reaches of East Anglia (north Norfolk) and the West Country (Gloucestershire) to find that minor piece of couture with the faded grandeur. Oh, the euphoria when she's spent hours rifling through smelly polyester to hit upon the Forties tea dress that fits like a dream. She's ecstatic, addicted and, the ultimate payback: cool – cool in the properly individual sense of the word. She's hit upon the true wisdom of style; she has cracked the code. She has just been given membership to the odd-looking elite of British style. Pass Go, collect £200 and get a subscription to *Cheap Date* magazine.

Everyone knows that designers find their inspiration from charity shops. The quality of the fabric is better and it's possible to learn a lot about construction and technique, which leads to the subject of making clothes. Before Punk hit the shops, Punks made their clothes by ripping, spraying and stencilling their 'normal' clothes. Buying a pattern from John Lewis, three metres of Liberty print and a zip can have a huge impact on a Miss E's style – and her sense of achievement. Even stitching together a piece of sari fabric from Brick Lane and buckling it up with a belt is an improvement on any generic clothing from Oxford Street. One step removed is to alter clothes picked up in charity shops: slashing hems, removing a collar, adding a row of big gold buttons. It's all in the detail. This is a most beautiful and practical part of Miss E's style education and having so much time to consider your outward personality never happens again.

Topshop has become a huge part of this stage, a bigger, more democratic version of an ideal Mary Quant set-up in the Sixties: fashion that is accessible and young. There is nothing better than a Saturday afternoon shared with like-minded teen spirits, carefully considering what your budget can stretch to. What must be avoided in these ready-outfit times is the bluffer's guide to style; in other words, an addiction to the high street where our heroine can fall prey to brainless cheap thrills. It takes time and effort to hone a unique style; it doesn't happen overnight, and here lies the danger of our quick-fix culture. The desire to have it all, right now, on credit, and preferably upgraded every week, has brought about, let's be honest here, a global style meltdown. What we need is a return to the personal reward of searching it out for yourself. But I am split here. The democratisation of style is vital to a non-elitist fashion Utopia, but it has also enforced the tyranny of the majority. Marketing has caught up with our honest eccentrics, exploited all their hard work – and flogged it for £9.99. Call me an old romantic.

But fear not. Miss E inherently knows how to use the high street and mix it up with the other, less obvious options. Most girls in this stage are desperate exhibitionists and deeply competitive. Their individuality must be protected at all costs; they would rather be seen dead than in something recognisable. 'Is that Primark?' 'God no, car boot,' she lies. She would sell her granny to get her hands on that vintage tweed Chanel jacket to mismatch with her one-off Japanese reissue, vintage, limited edition high-tops – nicked from her boyfriend. It's all about getting her hands on that one piece that sets her apart from the crowd and for this, the English style novice must put in the hours and get her hands dirty (literally – covered in a film of grime, the real stuff not a metaphor or a genre of music). No other nation spends so much time and effort dedicated to the grand old tradition of rummaging. *Cheap Date* – one of the greatest fanzines of all time – was devoted to just this; it was an ode to the artful car booter, the scavenger, the anti-fashion recessionista, all out there looking for that life-changing one-off.

Irony is significant at this stage of Miss E's progress. Sincerity is swapped for a sarcastic and wry take on the world; its idiosyncrasies can be explained by wit and double bluff. Getting it wrong is part of the process of getting it *right*. Her style is a satire, an intellectual referencing of what others term mistakes. Because *she's* wearing it, it's ironic. At this stage she can talk her way into and out of any style mishap. This is an important insight into English style.

In time, she will learn that too much irony can seriously

damage the romance of one's honest self-expression and can become a means of denying yourself things you actually really love just because you are afraid of being judged, but for now, while she's still working stuff out, it facilitates experimentation.

Of course, to be very fashionable, our recessionista avoids anything that *looks* fashionable. To the undiscerning eye, what she has on is just a T-shirt. To those in the know, its Heavy Metal band logo is as significant as her violet Marc Jacobs pumps (an eBay purchase), parka (picked up in New York) and (vintage) Gucci bag (thanks, mum). All tell of an interest in US hiphop, intelligent dance music, late Seventies R 'n' B and early Eighties soft rock. It's also called being pretentious. Self-deprecation and pretension form a wonderfully contrary juxtaposition. It's why all those girls and boys in bands stand pigeon-toed, looking like painful introverts while modelling glittery scarves, fluorescent catsuits and silver shoes. Get a load of me!

Oh, and this is another very important part of Miss E's stage three persona. Life will only be complete once she is in a band, or snagged a boyfriend who's the lead-singer of a band. Not your pop idol kind of ambition, you understand, but a true artistic yearning. Whether she's at St Martins or St Andrew's, the cool factor of standing at the side of a stage is unbeatable. In fact, a huge motivation for getting into higher education is the hope of finding her future soulmate/DJ/band members with the same visionary taste in gold lamé, oversized men's dinner jackets and ironic Eighties New Wave. So what if she doesn't know her A sharp from her B flat, she's come up with a great name, some existential lyrics and a deeply contrived image: it's going to inspire future generations!

Ultimately Miss E's style sense is defined by the decade of

her twenties: this Miss E won't hear a word against Bananarama. Just as mum with her kohl-lined eyes and pale lips is a Sixties girl at heart.

STAGE FOUR: PROPER JOB — If stage three is like going through a recession, then stage four is like suddenly finding a deep and totally bewildering affinity with the Thatcher years. Despite Mrs Thatcher's dubious legacy as prime minister (she thought being irresponsibly rich and middle class was okay), her penchant for big-shouldered calf-length skirt suits, silk pussy-bow blouses and handbags have secured her place among our most revered and stylish British birds.

And yet, despite the freedoms of her growing success and the sensory delights of luxury, it's a disconcerting time for our heroine. Her intense charity shop and high street training hasn't been forgotten. Yet the temptation to cast aside her frugal bent, to ignore thriftiness and embrace the world of designer purchases runs as deep as the need to drink the whole bottle of tequila. Miss E is trying to figure out where individuality fits in once she's passed through the gilded doors of Selfridges, or logged on to the perfect item minefield that is Net-A-Porter. This is our heroine's newest sartorial challenge. At this point, this monumental turning point in her life, she should probably head straight to the nearest Help the Aged shop and immerse herself in the comforting aroma of mothballs pungent with nostalgia and individuality. But the temptation to give in to the Pandora's box and submit to the power of Miu Miu is pretty damn impossible to resist.

Miss E has woken up to female empowerment. She is young enough to have a great body but old enough to earn a bit of disposable income. These are heady times. Shall I spend this month's wages on bills or buy the cheapest thing with a Goyard logo print I can find? Taking her hard-earned cash with a healthy pinch of innate sartorial flair and an eye for the ironic, she opts for expensive, witty purchases. Understanding the meaning and ideas behind her favourite designers is like being a teenager and aligning herself with a tribe; this is high art in the form of a skirt. At this stage in her seven ages there is only one god and her name is Rei Kawakubo and the place Miss E would happily die is in Dover Street Market. Here a lot of the contrary work is done for her; the merchandise has already been tested on the crash test dummies of sartorial style. It is a very safe place to take a first dip in the cool waters of designer names.

Suddenly Miss E is purchasing accessories, shoes, headbands and T-shirts at a quickening speed, aiming to buy into that brand that says everything her teenage tribe used to. She obsesses over the perfect item and reads hundreds of different theories and useless analytical nuances into this one rather clever bonded jacket. She has dressed it in so many different characters, put it with every conceptual idea in her wardrobe and WANTS IT. This jacket would change her life, her intellect, her friends, her boyfriend; no one could possibly question her as a human being if she had that jacket. She would wear it in a way that no one had ever thought of and the designer would probably take her, kiss her passionately and ask her to marry him and style his next show. This is obviously an extreme fantasy.

So she signs on to eBay. It becomes a Saturday morning swap-shop. It keeps her up at night. Here at the new trading floors of contemporary culture she buys and sells. At midnight she needs to outbid frankiefox66 by £3 – otherwise she will lose the vintage rattlesnake Hermès bag (so sick it has to be the ultimate statement). She types in the list of things she's looking for: Chanel lemon pumps (*très sportif*), Miu Miu wool camel bonded jacket, anything Balenciaga within reason, and waits for them to show up. She knows her top price but what she lacks in hard cash she makes up for in skill and commitment to the cause. But what does she do when she owns those things? She treats them as if they were her reviled school uniform, she customises, she flings on the floor; she wears them with anything that will dress them down. It is the equivalent of being embarrassed by a new best friend. There is something absolutely bloody marvellous and incredibly English about attaining that status symbol and then denying its status.

Another very special thing happens at this stage of Miss E's seven ages (as long as she has not veered from the true path of wisdom). She finds the *back room*. No VIP room in the world can compare to the back room of Rellik, the vintage store on Golborne Road. It takes time and energy for Miss E to work her way up the rails. The shop floor is now for the undergrads; the back room is where Miss E gains her Master's. It is no secret that half of Kate Moss's wardrobe once sat in these cramped quarters, which are the El Dorado of designer vintage. I remember the first time that the back half of Rellik was opened up to me; my coolest friend provided me with the all-important introduction, a knowing nod to the gatekeeper, Steve. I walked away with a Vivienne Westwood Pirate T-shirt dress and my personal Holy Grail – a sweater from the Westwood Witches collection bearing a design by Keith Haring.

There are, of course, the annoyingly privileged few who can bypass the demanding slog through charity shops and car boots. These distinguished Miss Es who have grannies who wore Balmain when it meant something, they get the true meaning of couture and luxury because they grew up surrounded by style – the style the great designers are looking to tap into. These lucky Miss Es develop a relaxed view of style – look at the ever-inspirational Dowager Duchess of Devonshire, who buys her clothes in Paris, at M&S and at agricultural shows – and that's it.

Yet, in retrospect, what every thirty-something doesn't miss is her twenty-something angst. The madness of love, the despair of heartbreak: it all leaves her tougher and wiser – and full of yearning. Miss E's twenties are a dizzy cycle of feeling cool, uncool, cool then uncool. Anxiety is exhausting. It's debilitating. Acutely conscious of being judged – of trying to fit in, she worries about not finding true love; she still goes clubbing but the crowd is starting to look half her age. She gets dumped by text and wakes up with a hangover.

Bring on 30.

STAGE FIVE: IT TAKES TWO — The day after her thirtieth birthday Miss England wakes up to the realisation that the trial of ticking boxes (room in a friend's house in London, tick, cripplingly expensive bag that now looks very old and filthy – great, tick. Small, badly paid job in the creative industries, extended work experience in magazines or publishing or cool transient non-job working for some unconventional aristo organising his archive, tick, DJ-ing at a Chanel party as the cool element, tick) is over. Hurrah. She has joined the semi-solvent-girl social demographic that thinks it invented stripped-floorboard-communal-living-with-novelty-coloured-walls (mine were dark purple).

At this point in my life, just before I was flung rather abruptly into motherhood, I was living in a large Victorian house in Ladbroke Grove – in cocooned chaos – owned by the lead-singer of Elastica and renowned rescuer of waifs and strays, Justine Frischmann. The third bedroom was occupied by Maya Arulpragasam, now the very famous M.I.A., another very stylish and rebellious female who made clothes out of brightly coloured fishnet tights. That girl loved colour. The house itself was typical of a contrary Miss E. It was a beautiful, Victorian house that had been randomly customised with rainbow painted stairs. A very low-lying corner sofa sat next to a huge record collection and set of decks; the kitchen table was covered in a film of ash and surrounded by people. The conservatory at the back was dominated by a Space Invaders machine. I loved that house, I loved my housemates and I loved my responsibility-free life. Life was about creating clothes, music, film, art, ideas, drama …

But while Miss E is now clever enough to help launch a friend's start-up magazine or blog (with a suitably clever, ironic title like *Fame*), master her downward dog (that's yoga or sex depending on her personal path of enlightenment), have dinner bought for her at the Wolseley, and obtain stage passes at Reading, she isn't clever enough to remember that if you don't use contraceptives you will have a baby.

Or did she want a baby? Happy accidents have worked up until now so why start to control it? Chaos works for clothes, why not for life – it's as good a theory as any in Miss E's universe. Just as her style taste is taking on PhD status, life comes and hits her in the face. Oh, how cruel. Oh, how great.

On the morning that she eats four fry-ups in her favourite greasy spoon and still feels hungry – pretending it's an irreverent lifestyle choice as opposed to abject gluttony – she heads to Boots. Ah, Boots. Entering the chemist is a nostalgia trip that takes her back to nicking her first eyeliner and now here she is, with her Boots points card, buying a pregnancy test. Boots has been a friend to her throughout her journey. Boots is a classless monument to English culture. She loves Boots. She cries in Boots.

That evening, sitting on the loo, she watches the line turn blue. She looks at her icons pasted all over the deep purple bathroom walls and they look back at her through their irresponsible drug-addled hazes, and reality kicks in. This isn't a game any more. Her humour fades as the sense of amazement that her body is doing what her body *should* do is matched by a fear that travels right to the heart of her: fear of global warming, fear of motherhood, fear of getting fat, fear of the natural order. Her boyfriend-of-six-weeks doesn't mention wedding bells but suggests buying a car, an old, battered Volvo. This appeals. She takes it as a 'Yes, I Want to Be a Dad' and the decision is thus made for her. Miss E will now become a mother and so the cycle of life moves on.

So far, so in keeping with life's formal plan. But where's the twist and how did life's formal plan catch up with Miss E? Never fear. Her innate sense of perverse taste will see her through this one as it has faithfully done up until now.

Pregnancy doesn't stop her thinking about clothes or her image. Pregnancy is actually very good for budding eccentrics. It offers an interesting sartorial challenge. (Note to self: Neneh Cherry is a very good role model for a kind of Buffalo Girl-style bump.) Yet right now our heroine is feeling pretty uncertain about what her body is going to do next – and where her life is heading. This is where boyfriend dressing really comes into its own. She raids her boyfriend's cupboards, again, and wears his old T-shirts, jeans and oversized dinner jackets. Those Iggy Pop

T-shirts (whose mother, by the way, was called Luella – just had to get that in somewhere) that were just the wrong side of oversized before, now work perfectly. There's not a flowing boho dress in sight, phew. Instead, the emotions of motherhood are given a casual male confidence that she needs – mixing androgyny with the ultimate feminine statement – procreation in skinny jeans.

At John Lewis a matronly lady with a tape measure tells her that she will be a 38E by the time she is full-term (is that the same as Jordan?). She fits Miss E for her first pregnancy bra; a tricky look stylistically. It is a well-known fact that clothes hang better without the hindrance of boobs. That, anyway, is the accepted view of male designers and one that has somehow morphed into her personal view. She can see clearly now (the rain has gone). She is a woman without a desperate desire for a pre-pubescent boy's body. Embracing motherhood is the first truly rebellious thing she has ever done in her life. What's more, the bra is the sort her granny wore. Is this a subversive style message? There has to be a frumpy Prada element somewhere, or is this purely pragmatic? Bugger that – Agent Provocateur do it all for you with a leopard print breastfeeding bra – is nothing sacred?

Then comes the baby and the party stops. Life is suddenly very hard with hormonal mood swings, cracked nipples that even the AP bra can't abate and the utterly hideous sleep-deprivation. What happened to spending hours pontificating over that particular day's outward character? The world of runny faeces and milk and vomit can be a dark, macabre place. But it doesn't matter, you see, because from this chaos comes a sense of completeness, authenticity if you will, that she had imagined might be out there but had no idea where. This is it. This *is* life. And love.

And with this sense of self comes a truer understanding of her Englishness. She is finally beginning to emulate the legend that is the pragmatic, stuff-and-nonsense British matriarch, while still effortlessly retaining the eyeliner that has been growing steadily more smudged through complete neglect of personal grooming (which has just reached new Patti Smith heights, along with an extreme version of matted bed hair). Grunge has never been so appropriate.

A few months later and they are standing in a field. The fantasy becomes even more fully imagined. She can create a new eccentric ethereal persona. The pagan naming ceremony (complete with white witch) gives her some much-needed English castle-in-the-sky. She finds a Seventies folk number in Virginia's in Holland Park – it's very Britt Ekland in *The Wicker Man* – and there is a distinct possibility of a similar fertility dance later on in a bid to reclaim her stylish past and create a new fantastical character roughly based on herself but much, much more interesting.

But, just as she's got the hang of it, simultaneously breast-feeding and sending emails, it's time to go back to work. (There's a knack to multi-tasking while breastfeeding, believe me. I've breastfed my kids in the weirdest places, the weirdest being an executive meeting at Target world headquarters in Minnesota. They obviously thought I was a quaint, rather peculiar London girl and breastfeeding was just another one of my anarchic quirks so hey, bring it on.)

Eighteen months later and, holy shit, the stick turns blue again – must have been that naked fertility dance – powerful stuff that paganism. Must stop reading all that occult literature. Miss E should probably go back to contraception school for a few basic lessons but, as you can see, she is now working against life's formal plan. She decides not to go back to work at all; she would rather be there for the kids, *enjoy* her time with them and drop out to become the bohemian vegetable garden anarchist she always secretly wanted to be. (Move over Debo Mitford, there's a new duchess in town and she feeds her chickens in Christopher Kane.) What is it about English women and gardening?

What fate lies ahead? One of mediocrity and boredom? Bump back to earth, oh shit, of course I don't have a bloody garden, I live in London. Will our heroine turn into a neurotic Wendy Craig in the Eighties sitcom *Butterflies*, burning the fish fingers and flirting with a dark-haired stranger? Mind you, Wendy had a good look with those swirly patterned blouses, A-line skirts and pussy-bow shirts, so perhaps it wouldn't be so bad after all, minus the adultery.

STAGE SIX: BACK IN THE SADDLE — Before the sixth stage of Miss England's progress can begin, the really tough first few years of childcare have to be done. Those are the lost years, when mind and body are placed in the service of a higher cause – when Miss E resembles a barren fashion wasteland, with tumbleweed and nondescript pieces of shapeless clothing blowing through her ghost town of a wardrobe, when all that remains of her style is an allegiance to grungy oversized plaid shirts and a pair of obligatory skinny jeans that aren't looking their best. Only once that's all over can stage six begin – and with it, she can finally get back to the important job of statement dressing. But the statements she's now making are much more profound, because she is different; into that mix of naive irony and rebellion has been thrown one huge bit of life experience. That childcare time wasn't lost by any means – it was a time of self-discovery, of reality-checking, with a down-at-heel charm that's deepened her. That self-deprecation could easily have turned into self-annihilation, but that last bout of self-scrutiny is the last, most vicious lesson before enlightenment arrives.

Now she's back in the saddle though, and the sixth stage is one of deep thought and scrutiny, paring everything down to the bare essentials. Life in her twenties was responsibility-free, self-indulgent and fun – but her overconfident outfit choices looked as though they were wearing her, as if being on, ahead of and subverting trends was all that really mattered. In her thirties, just as she's shedding her inhibitions and neuroses, she's also shedding pretentiousness and mixed references. Not every stage of life is about trawling through dens of iniquity to find that pair of Eighties plastic sunglasses that define you. There's angst a plenty in your forties, but trying to clothe oneself in edgy apparel starts to seem small fry when compared to grown-up stuff like feeding your family and trying to leave your legacy to the world before it's too late.

With all of life's big distractions, and attempting to grow up, the thirties and forties are when a Miss E starts to think about putting the frivolous side of outward expression behind her (this is only ever partially successful, as eccentricity is in her life-blood, after all). By the late thirties and early forties, things have really begun to change, and this is when questions about the real essence of her being and what looks best on her come together. She begins to base her dressing-up decisions on who *she* is; she knows how to complement what she's feeling. She wonders: does this greying, threadbare T-shirt really sum up the complexities of my personality? The paring down and the thoughtfulness only go so far though – she would still rather die than dress 'correctly' in the French way, and being contrary, intentionally wrong and throwing something really ugly in there all still feels like part of her birthright.

Sensible and boring though the sixth age might seem, it's the moment when your inner character starts to make sense – and you start to dress as the person you actually are. It's when you look for clothes that enhance your idiosyncrasy and grown-up sex appeal. Looking like the person you are – a believable character – is about making small, careful and clever adjustments. (A friend of mine has just started wearing braces with everything, which gives a slight change in her proportions, which seems to say something new and exciting about her style.) Personal style is now a matter of bringing out the real substance of yourself, not creating a superficial image. This is the stage I'm arriving at now – a stage of horror, relief and confidence, all in equal parts.

With her new, more restrained eccentricity there's a new attention on the cleverly contrived details – the precise kind of fabric, the toe-shape of the shoes (not round but not pointed – like the perfect toes of Miss Philo's Celine collection – that's a British bird who has this stage down to a fine art). Everything now means something – the length of a shirt collar sheds light on the person she has become. The cleverness is in the ratio of out-there to conservative – that's where her stylish experience and superiority shine through. For Miss E, her new subtlety can come in the shape of a twenty-by-ten-inch hair bow worn with a crisp man's shirt, a pair of perfectly indigo jeans and a Hermès belt. For those now whispering claims to sartorial (and satirical) perfection – as opposed to screaming out individuality in as many mismatched, in-joke statement pieces as she can get her hands on – accessories are devilishly important. Finding the right kind of accessories is now tricky – but Miss E has a solid grounding in all things eccentric, traditional and rebellious. She's done flea markets, department stores, high street, provincial farmers' markets, and all the boutiques and car boots and boyfriends' and friends' wardrobes in-between.

By the sixth age, her new tendency for paring down sees Miss E buying lots of things that look very similar – be those army shirts, fisherman's sweaters, varying degrees of a very particular shade of denim, shoulderpads, minis and maxis. Many of them are signs of the years that matter to her – my favourite personal time warp is skinny jeans and sloppy cardis (Grunge).

Another development of the sixth age is her attitude to fabrics – the fabrics a young Miss E used to buy without a second feel start to grate, and they cling annoyingly to a more mature chassis. She starts to prefer the posh stuff, and a clever cut becomes a necessity for practical reasons, not just because of some style theory. Not that a good cut has to mean boring – an extreme shoulder or an alternative moulded shape is still, to a more worldly character, worthy of exploration. There's still room for satire and irony, but Miss E wants her clothes to be well made, and they need to have more about them than a well-informed and clever but fashion-world allusion. There are fewer instantly gratifying Saturday night purchases in bad quality silk, and polyester mixes enter the hallowed halls of her wardrobe/bedroom floor rarely. (Yes, Miss E still has slobbish tendencies.) Now, luxury wool jackets and high-waisted black tuxedo trousers litter the area around her bed.

Right now, this particular Miss E feels a strong synergy with traditional English factories – caring about craftsmanship makes her a continuing part of English tradition. Carefully crafted details render her special; she sits comfortably among her English tribe but she has a unique personal style that has come from years of personal honing and experimentation.

Quality hasn't had too much importance before – suddenly it's quality over quantity every time and expensive footwear becomes, inexplicably, rational. After years of study our heroine has refined her art. She can spot a dubious, seasonal designer reference at twenty paces (well, most of the time) – the sixth age Miss E prefers the classics or the genuinely original, although, it being her determined approach, she'll still wear them with something that throws them out in the wrong direction.

Miss E has now gained the upper hand and has wrestled free from the control of 'how to look cool'. She has started to wear the clothes – she is in charge of them, not the other way round. Now this can go two ways; it can mean embracing the freedom to be a bit silly and more experimental – think of the genius Helena Bonham-Carter, who hints at the final stage of the seven ages, Granny Nirvana, or the late Isabella Blow – or it can mean finding your inner chic and not being afraid to look your age. But there is a big question here and it's to do with how much irony you are honestly applying. How long before the established English tradition – and its frumpery – that you are mocking becomes the very thing that you are? At what point have you been doing something ironically for so long that there's no longer any irony in it, and, when you ask yourself, you find that you're just doing it straight, with no irony at all? It's a question I often try to get my head round as I ask myself – honestly – how much irony there really is in my current choices of country casual tweeds, straight leg jeans and court shoes (thank God for the English condition of scruffy hair and bitten nails). You wonder if the joke just might be on you, as your studied conformity and conservative outfits seem less and less witty and more of an honest reflection of what you've become – a middle-aged woman with a hankering for lost rebellion. Yes, it really happens; behind

your love of all things contrary, you discover you're quietly meta-
morphosing into your mother. Middle age is a disconcerting but
life-affirming time.

STAGE SEVEN: GRANNY NIRVANA —

Stage seven of Miss England's progress means … stop thinking
and start playing. The rationality and sagacity of stage six is behind her, now it's time to have a bit of a laugh. British grannies
do this better than anyone else. To get the obvious out of the
way: being an English granny does have its downside. Deterio-
ration and decay are inevitable and sure to occupy one's mind on
occasion. But to set against that there's a colossal new freedom.
This gives English grannies their cracking sense of humour, not
to mention a genius wardrobe. At last you have the freedom to
be whoever the bugger you want – whatever path an English
granny takes, it is as uncompromising as when she was a toddler
in her mother's pearls, only with marginally more bad language,
a lot more worldliness and a practical approach to life's intrica-
cies. There's a defiant pragmatism, a brilliant logic and a fuck-it
insouciance to my favourite grannies. I'll sum up their thinking
as: 'So what if I'm grumpy, I'm allowed to be. So what if I'm fat,
I'm allowed to be, I'm old!' There are no limits to the amount of
blue eyeshadow and pink lipstick a seventh-stage Miss E might
apply – maybe with a slightly shaky hand – after all, it's up to her.
   Just look at the brilliant, uncompromising, no-nonsense
grannies we have. Something of what I admire is summed up in
Catherine Tate's 'Gran', a machine-gun of expletives and vulgar-
ity with wrinkly tan tights and a killer smoker's cackle, and also
there's Vanessa Redgrave, the pinnacle of over-seventy chic, with
an experienced but elegant face and lots of fluid black clothing

and costume jewellery. We've got Vita Sackville-West – an androgynous intellectual with a progressive sense of morality – Marianne Faithfull (rock goddess), Vivienne Westwood (make-up caked experimentalist) and the Queen (a gun-toting, ruddy-faced, head-scarfed countryside-lover). Then there's Agatha Christie, such a sweet be-tweeded little old lady who likes Earl Grey in Royal Doulton and a good murder mystery, but we know that she knows all the awful secrets.

By this seventh stage, our Miss E has seen and done everything. She has been through every incarnation of rebellion, anarchy, subversion, conformity, tribal affiliation, bad haircuts, irony, apathy, and has arrived at total freedom of expression. She has spent a lifetime tailoring her looks to express changing personal manifestos – some embarrassing, some witty, some cool, some geeky, some sincere and some ironic. Editing her style for chosen members of the opposite sex or work environments, or anything that may have hindered and closeted her style desires – it's all in the past. Now she can be single-minded and any tribal allegiance is limited to the Women's Institute (and what a sublime group of style leaders they are). She has dignity, and it's because she has weathered the storms of life. Now she has achieved wisdom and can be completely herself – everything has been leading to this heady moment.

Now the fun can be put back into dressing up (or down, or sideways). If a seventh-stager looks like a batty old eccentric, or chooses to wear hats again and match them to handbags and shoes, well, why the hell not? My most cherished granny look is the most pragmatic – wear all your biggest sweaters at once and some woolly socks over your tights to save on the heating, a comfortable pair of shoes, a nice comfy elasticated-waist skirt, a headscarf to keep your set in place (or a good fur hat if your hairstyle allows it) and a good rain mac and carry a brolly at all times. Oh, and a good sturdy shopper or a carrier bag to keep all your essential items in. Some of this thoroughly British look might be down to the crap weather and dubious welfare system, and it's sometimes accompanied by too much Lily of the Valley. Sometimes it almost becomes a self-parody – but it's a beautiful one.

The glorious, who-cares, pile-it-on granny style – and grandad's can be pretty rousing too – is continually inspiring me, because for this Miss E there is nothing quite so worrying as looking fashionably correct, with all choices dictated by designers. If the street is where Miss E will find her style *A-to-Z*, grannies are the unbeatable expression of the eccentricity that's the key to true English style. Elsewhere in the world, style is now often hindered by neurotic attempts at youthfulness and the thread has been lost (apart, that is, from the surgeon's thread). If a dark and weak moment catches you – predictably – thinking about wrinkles, consider how sexy Marianne Faithfull is: wrinkles maketh the ultimate, stylish expression of a life lived with sartorial grace and tribal history. A granny also knows better than everyone else how to make-do-and-mend, which is something any true Miss E grows to understand too.

Grannies are the queens of the exuberant mismatch, the guardians of the idea that to really know about style you also have to know that it isn't about rules or strictness, it's about expressing yourself in a way you feel comfortable with, without the need for clever nuance or subtext. This very English idea can, though, seem flummoxing abroad. A rather grand French fashion editor once exasperatedly asked: 'What is it wiz zees English girls? Why do zey insist on zis ugly dressing?' To which the answer is simple – *because* it's wrong!

THE
BRITISH BOSOM:
SOME VARIETIES

—

THE SHELF — The mature English filly with womanly curves hoists her ample bosom up and then compresses it – with the aid of a supremely cantilevered Rigby & Peller bra – thereby creating a shelf. The shelf lies beneath her buttoned-up blouse – Jaeger, Hardy Amies or NHS standard issue – like a dormant volcano; on the surface the shelf expresses supreme calm and eternal firmness, but its powerful femininity can mean only one thing – that beneath the shelf womanly feelings rage.

The Queen, our Royal matriarch, epitomises comforting maternal instincts and matronly authority, with a strong dash of royal munificence thrown into the mix. The Queen's shelf always remains resolute in the face of possible disaster, whether she is riding a horse, reviewing the forces or quietly handing Rich Teas to the corgis. Princess Anne and late-arrival-to-the-royal-ranks Camilla are also staunch proponents of the shelf. Princess Di would eventually have opted for the shelf, but in her short-lived prime preferred to get them out; they spilled out of her taffeta gowns in a most unroyal way and thereby went some way to modernising a reluctant monarchy.

THE SHELF WITH FLAN ON DISPLAY — Beneath a jumper – close-fitting for the bold – the shelf is just a shelf: a jutting, proud statement of womanly virtue and the passion that might be raging beneath. But with a lower cut dress – and maybe a more uplifting bra – the shelf is elevated to become a display cabinet for what Tom Wolfe has described as 'flan'. This is a particularly English display, easily recognisable in any costume drama film, and at Saturday night dinner parties in rural vicarages; the display of flan indicates a forthright yet innocently uncomplicated method of showing off one's assets. (The flan is the sworn enemy of the fake boob and would shudder at finding itself in such company.) Here I defer to the distinguished flâneur Mr Wolfe. I think he was the first to use the term 'flan' in this way in his 1968 story, 'The Life and Hard Times of A Teenage London Society Girl':

> This dress Sue has on she went to Portobello Road and bought it second-hand, in one of those shops. It is made of mandarin-orange velvet, with the hem about five inches above the knees and the bodice low and cut straight across with just straps over the shoulder, with the upper parts of her breasts showing like two trembling servings of flan.

THE TWO FRIED EGGS — Kate Moss, the antithesis of the airbrushed, interchangeable celebrity, has never shied from getting her kit off. When she does, the world is greeted by the sight of her perfectly formed chest – feminine but tomboyish, and real. When France was entranced by Brigitte Bardot, Twiggy was the champion of the girlish, rather than the womanly, figure – beginning a happy English love affair with the smaller bosom (Sarah Lucas joked about this in her 1996 painting *Self Portrait with Fried Eggs*). Very few girls manage to hang on to their bra-less tits for ever. With babies comes milky engorgement, which usually leads to a permanent change in proportion. However, in a particular twist of fate, a well-endowed bosom post-babies can revert to two fried eggs.

MILITANT MAMMORIES — Planting the baby on the table, lactating mum rummages inside her vintage Chloe shirt before plonking her breastfeeding boobs out on the table. She shoves a squirting nipple into her son's mouth with agricultural flourish. At his birthday party, he runs over and pulls out a boob to suckle before racing back to finish his chocolate brownie. She knows she shouldn't allow her son to maul her, he's *two* years old for God's sake, but it's so hard because he's *so* adorable. 'Bitty' has paraded over-age breastfeeding for the English phenomenom it really is – the *Little Britain* character that has horrified the nation is not so far away from the truth. Bitty does have a rather drastic effect on one's boobs but the British woman can turn this into a style statement of rebellious practicality with hippy undertones, and dress it in a really good vintage dress.

BIRDS OF
BRITAIN:
A GUIDE

—

Be wicked, be brave, be drunk,
be reckless, be dissolute, be despotic,
be an anarchist ... be anything you
like, but for pity's sake be it to the top
of your bent. Live – live fully, live
passionately, live disastrously.

VITA SACKVILLE-WEST

The British bird is as recognisable as the Queen. And one only
needs to look at the older members of the monarchy to know
that sartorial eccentricity is alive and well. (Here I should apol-
ogise for muddling Englishness and Britishness; I'm actually
writing about English style but I'm going to use artistic licence
to generalise and lump them together for the sake of argument.
Scotland, Wales and Ireland all have a similarly contrary aesthetic and attitude. When it comes to style we are united and all
clothing and traditional costume is fair game.)

We could start by considering what the British bird has given
the world. Bestriding the globe like an overconfident little girl
dressed up in her mother's (and father's) clothes, in shoes and
blazers that are too big, and jeans that are too tight and short
and hair that is a peculiar shade of washed-out weird and a bit
limp, she is a genuine oddball. She is creative, witty, fearless,
pioneering, curious, sharp, contrary, rebellious, nonchalantly
wrong and, above all, original. In common with our weather, you
can never be completely sure what you're going to get. Now
there's a lot to be said for taking a conventional approach to things
– and adding a twist. It derives in part from irony and the English sense of humour, but also from our intellectual superiority.

The upper-class sense of entitlement *plus* working-class tribalism and middle-class questioning *equals individualism*. My unruly flock with their mass of contradictions – and their tempestuous private lives – epitomise the zeal, the uncompromising attitude, and above all the spirit that lies at the heart of English style. They are representative of a certain type of female disobedience. I'm thinking of Barbara Hulanicki, aged 73, in black nail varnish, Vita Sackville-West in a man's trilby and long strings of pearls. Their feigned indifference to the power of their feminine and masculine charms (androgyny is integral to their style) is a ruse to overturn the rules. But don't be fooled. Cool detachment is a British bird's strength.

The collective experience and ideas of these British birds span a century and remain influential. They are inspirational. Yet on writing this, I feel a tide of outrage at all those British birds who aren't properly recognised for their contribution to cultural life, which is why I've included a few runners-up.

I WANT BLUE PLAQUES FOR ALL MY
B I R D S — Vita's legacy, the gardens at Sissinghurst and her prodigious output of books, has been a call to respect the land and preserve the past. The same could be said of the Duchess of Devonshire, the last of the Mitford sisters. When she goes so will a part of England, along with her gossipy essays on life at Chatsworth – best served hot with buttered crumpets and a pot of Earl Grey tea.

Vivienne Westwood, early in her career, made the point that sex is funny and provocation is crucial; so are English dress codes. Her trick has been to connect divergent narrative styles with humour and intelligence and turn them into something new (aristos in platforms, cowboys in tweed). This knack of combining tradition and innovation is a feature common to all my British birds. Sixties style icon Jane Ormsby-Gore was an original Portobello girl, mixing vintage with couture and subverting the conventions she was born into.

I realise that I'm painting with a very broad brush – but that might be the way to paint these greatest of birds, who, whatever they stand for in life, all handed something new to English style. Mrs Thatcher turned the handbag from a noun into a verb; brash poet Lily Allen has become synonymous with Chanel, that international symbol of luxury and wealth, which has probably led to howls of anguish at the Palais Royal. PJ Harvey, another singer-songwriter, has avoided the trap of wearing what she as a celebrity is told to wear. Instead, she has struck out with her own deviant originality intact, in sequins, catsuits, Forties-style bathing costumes, horrific beauty queen make-up and Gothic black, using her style to strengthen her thought-provoking character. My birds are striking for the interpretive manner in which they have redefined English style. Mary Quant put youth on the fashion map. Paula Yates's Fifties dresses became *her* means of self-expression – and were so seditiously feminine at a time when masculine tailoring and nylon shell suits had a stranglehold on English dress codes.

Kate Moss is self-taught, a perfectionist and the mistress of her craft. She's never short of ideas and has a passion for character, evidenced by the timeless appeal of her Sixties rock chick meets naive scruffy girl in customised T-shirts. Her style is the most naturally synchronistic with her spirit.

British birds are the power behind the throne; their romps through the last century live on in the adventures of today's generation of truly diverse British girls. I see their exploits as part pantomime, part guerrilla warfare and I've sought to recreate the wit and mayhem of their lives in my collections.

Just a small aside though – compiling this list of birds has been a nightmare. It's taken me months of deliberation and then I would stupidly show my list of birds to someone who would violently disagree. However, in the end these women are inspiring to me. For this very personal list I chose each for their originality, individuality, spirit and inherent Englishness.

The runners-up and the top ten have been changed and changed back, promoted, demoted, overlapped and some people have been completely missed out. Forgive me – make up your own – send all candidates to the above address. One other thing – this is not a best-dressed list. These birds are more than mere clothes horses. It's all in the attitude, dear reader.

I still have sleepless nights over those commendable birds that are too rare to be spotted.

BRITISH BIRDS — RUNNERS-UP

THE QUEEN — Hats *orf* to Her Majesty for refusing to submit to the tyranny of spurious fashion trends. The Queen reigns as the original revivalist, refusing to deviate from a style developed in the Fifties but tweaking it ever so slightly in order to remain just this side of eccentric. The Queen is a courageous pioneer of head-to-toe lemon. There are not many who could carry that one *orf*.

AGATHA CHRISTIE — Tweed skirts, furs, brooches, sensible shoes, thick stockings, pearls, horn-rimmed glasses – and murder most foul – make Ms Christie an indomitable force for good in the traditional style stakes. My good friend Katie Grand first opened my eyes to the genius of Christie, making me watch copious amounts of episodes while pointing out the subtle interplay of calf length and pleated skirts (she was working with Miuccia Prada at the time).

BARBARA HULANICKI — The co-founder of Sixties fashion boutique Biba – a store that grew and grew until one day it found itself towering over Kensington as a rather ironic, brilliant and satirical take on a traditional department store. Barbara was and is a natural rebel, wearing twin sets the wrong way round with the buttons at the back – and chopping up shoes. We English girls just love chopping things up. It's a rite of passage for any Miss England worth their domestic sewing machine and Hulanicki was a riotous preacher on the subject.

She started making clothes out of necessity and became the holder of the keys to a retro fantasy in which feather boa'd girls wandered through fields in maxi-dresses. This later became

PLATE NO. 2 ∗ THE QUEEN

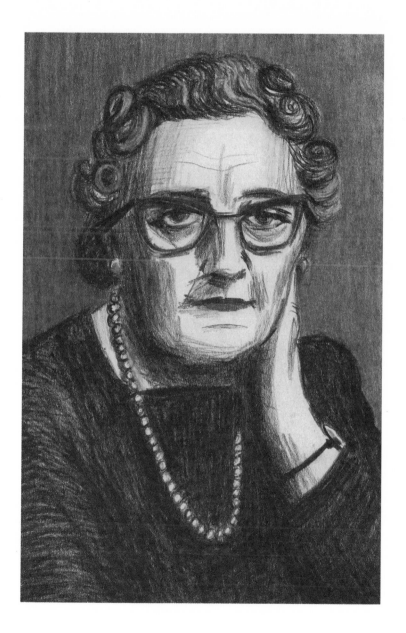

PLATE NO. 3 * AGATHA CHRISTIE

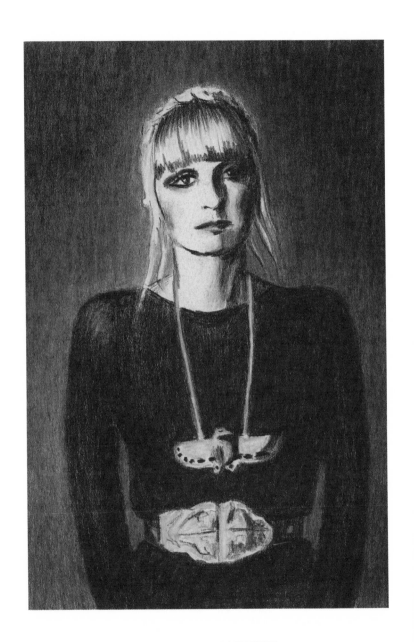

PLATE NO. 4 * BARBARA HULANICKI

known as Seventies British Romanticism (joined by Laura Ashley and Ossie Clark) but she always gave it an edge and a sense of fun. I for one am astonished by the genius of putting Biba Baked Beans alongside some of the most desirable dressing-up clothes on the planet.

Hulanicki, in her seventies, is still producing work – she recently did a collection for Topshop, and produced my favourite fashion book ever, *In Biba* (there is also another great one called *SinBiba*), written by Delisia Howard and illustrated by Barbara and C Price. It's a modern graphic romance/fairy tale, the delirious story in poetry and pictures of a girl who started a shop and made girls smile, scream, self-combust, self-style and become disciples of said girl, shop and consequent lifestyle.

Like all brilliant and iconic ventures, Biba crashed and burned and Barbara lost the rights to the name. It is the only way to go: make fashion fast, kill it before anyone gets bored – therefore guaranteeing cult status. They – those with the cash – tried to resurrect Biba not so long ago. I even got a call to see if I wanted to do it, but you simply can't mess with a label that was so much about its creator. Biba was a glorious moment in time and only one woman could make Biba work.

I recently did a fashion tent at a festival with Ms Hulanicki, making cocktail dresses out of wallpaper and tinfoil at the rebellious, stately Port Eliot. It felt like one of those projects that really was making everyday things that can change your life – one of the key tenets of her book – at least, it made everyone happy. I was honoured that she chose me to do it with her. She really is an original rebel and made me think what fashion is all about.

ANNABELLA LWIN — Long before heiress Punk Alice Dellal shaved her head, 14-year-old – yes, 14 – Annabella-with-a-Mohican pogo-ed on to the stage as the singer with Bow Wow Wow (African-beats-Balinese-chanting-girlish-squealing). She was immortalised topless, looking over her shoulder, in a pastiche of Manet's *Le Déjeuner sur l'herbe* – shot for a Bow Wow Wow record cover. She ruled the charts as the nouveau Punk girl in the vintage tulle dresses.

SIOUXSIE SIOUX — Emerging from the male clamour of Punk with her dark, ethereal, Geisha Punk looks and deep howl, Siouxsie Sioux – like Westwood – cut a tomboyish figure. Hers was a melancholy anger, from a glowering but romantic hard-nut who probably hung out by night in graveyards drinking gin. By 1978 with the success of 'Hong Kong Garden', she had created a Gothic, theatrical stage persona that included fishnet tights, keffiyehs, emblazoned T-shirts, men's shirts, hot-pants and a hell of a lot of black – a kind of romantic dominatrix. And in doing so she inspired a whole new breed of darker, witchier, more feeling Punks. She took the anarchy of Punk and made it artful and theatrical, her hands – gloved in black lace – and sharp black fingernails dramatically encircling her lily-white face and framing her exquisitely terrifying make-up. The ultimate rock chick, she never lost her feline elegance. Her music always teetered on that most enchanting of brinks, that between the violently tough and the fragile but beautiful.

ISABELLA BLOW — Isabella had all the qualities of some dark female protagonist lurking heroically in a strange English novel written by a Mitford, and transformed into animation by Tim Burton. She was dark, fragile, ugly and beautiful at the same

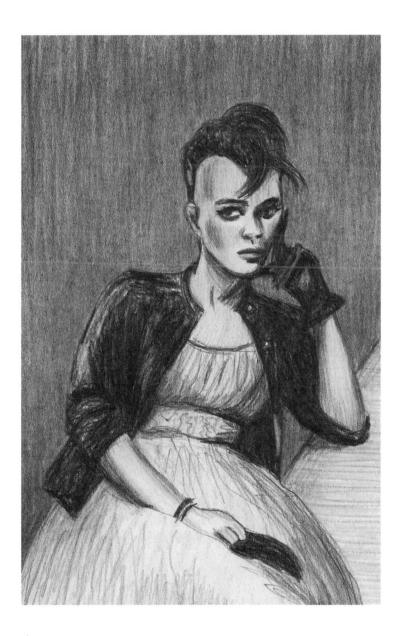

61

BIRDS OF
BRITAIN:
A GUIDE

PLATE NO. 5 * ANNABELLA LWIN

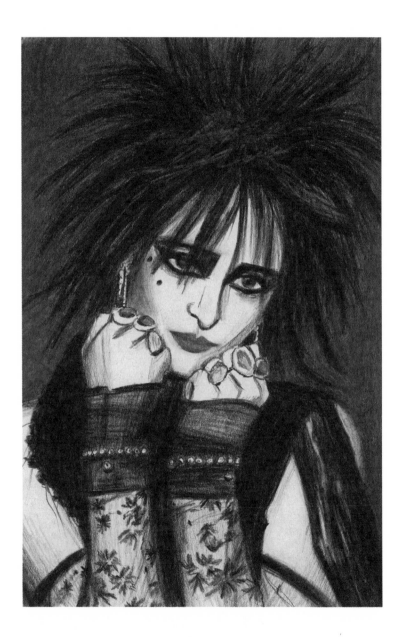

PLATE NO. 6 ∗ SIOUXSIE SIOUX

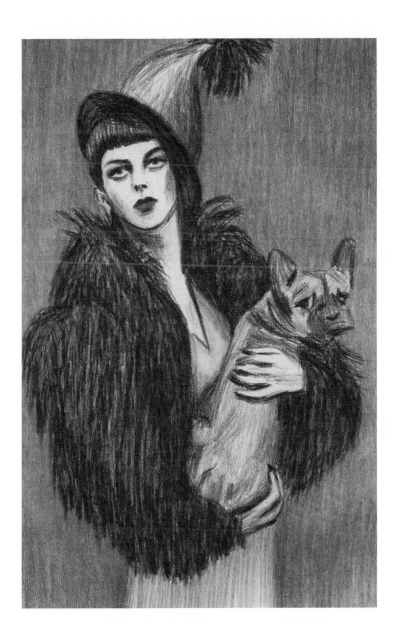

PLATE NO. 7 • ISABELLA BLOW

time. English to the core, passionate beyond anything, she lived in a fantastical tragedy of love, murder, suicide and overwhelming emotion. She was totally overemotional, utterly kind to those who ignited her imagination, vehemently vile to those she found depressingly dull. She was typical in her aristocratic traits – intimidating and deeply insecure at all times – and a product of the conflict between her traditionalism and complete nihilism.

There are many of her kind in the fashion world – posh birds who love a bit of working-class designer-genius totty. Harlech, Guinness, Ferry, all outwardly confident, upper-class eccentrics fighting over the ownership of the McQueens and the Gallianos of this world. Blow was the ultimate patron, who wore her love and emotion for everyone to see, even if covered by a hat of gargantuan proportions and concept.

She hid herself away and was an exhibitionist, all at the same time. She talked about love incessantly and she nurtured to the point of obsession the people she applauded and mothered – from Alexander McQueen to Stella Tennant.

A devoted Miss England, she didn't give a crap as long as people made a 'bloody effort'. She died, tragically, by drinking weed killer; even her death was a statement of English eccentricity.

AMY WINEHOUSE — Conflict, tragedy, vulnerability, creativity and rebellion – there is a pattern forming here – you don't have to have self-destruction in your very being to be in this list, but it helps. But this compilation is about style lest we forget and Amy's style is unique. Hers is a conflict that, ultimately, looks achingly and sublimely considered. She is dishevelled and high-maintenance in equal parts, and both parts are equally extreme and cartoonish in proportion.

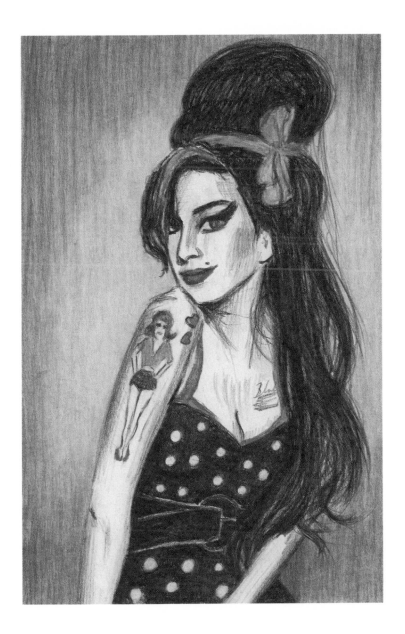

PLATE NO. 8 * AMY WINEHOUSE

The Billie Holiday pencil skirts, the gingham shirts, the fitted, corseted, belted, Betty Boop dresses – all boobs and hips and calves, coupled with that dance, tightly controlled in its abandon and occasional drunken stumble. And the icing on the cake is, of course, the mountainous beehive with its cute polka dot bow, a scarf or the name of her beau embedded halfway up. Then the sailor tattoos that just make her look even sexier – neutralising the cute and rendering her sex appeal rather dangerous, as if she would scratch like her beloved cat.

It's as if she's lost in her passion for the music and lifestyle of her heroines. This is a genuine passion, not the neat re-working of a retro sound and look. It's as if Ella Fitzgerald and Billie Holiday have possessed her. Her life, her music and her style are love letters to those women and those times but to their spirit she also adds her own tortured talent. She is not so much influenced by their work as she is an extension of the period, writing with honest poetry of the darkness of passion and of love.

Amy screams of sultry sex but in an innocent, girl-dressing-up-in-heels kind of a way (her death-defying heels always look a size too big, adding to the vulnerability of her shuffling dance moves). 'I don't listen to anyone except my inner child,' said Amy. A cross between a kind of warped Barbie and Sid Vicious, her talent for songwriting and dressing and self-destruction is raw, unique and genuinely from the heart.

She is the only girl who managed to bring the besequinned flower dress from my spring–summer 2008 Batman collection to life, making it look sexy, retro and tough. The dress got caught up in her character and liked it (she thumped someone while wearing it at Glastonbury – a defining moment for that dress).

JANE ORMSBY-GORE — Born into a traditional upper-class English family, Jane 'came out' in 1960 in fluffy, puffy white tulle – and vowed never to wear it again. She soon set about cutting up jeans from America to make hipsters, slashing skirts into minis and wearing second-hand clothes from the Chelsea Antique and Portobello markets.

In 1966 her then husband Michael Rainey opened Hung on You, a Chelsea men's boutique that sold leather jerkins and Byron shirts with frilly fronts and big sleeves, handmade by East End tailors. Jane was the brains behind the clothes that dressed the Rolling Stones (who titled their song 'Lady Jane' after her) and the Beatles. 'You did have to dig about in antique shops,' she said. 'I remember finding a shoe buckle with huge great emeralds, all paste with fake jewels … which now everybody wears all the time.'

MARGARET THATCHER — Mrs T was the original Eighties power-dresser but she began public life as a very different type of blonde.

The year was 1972 … The BBC TV cameras were ready to roll. At the last possible minute, a group of men in dark suits ushered in a blonde woman wearing floor-length scarlet chiffon, with ice-blue stones winking at earlobes and throat. This glamour puss was the secretary of state for education in Edward Heath's government.

A few months later she was advised to tone down her look (was that the moment it all went so politically wrong, when she lost her chiffon?) and she went on to become the scary lady who ran the country for 13 years. The look she did it in included big-shouldered calf-length skirt suits from Aquascutum in navy or sapphire (occasionally checked tweed), Marks & Spencer pussy-bow shirts, the ubiquitous pearls and round-toed Salvatore

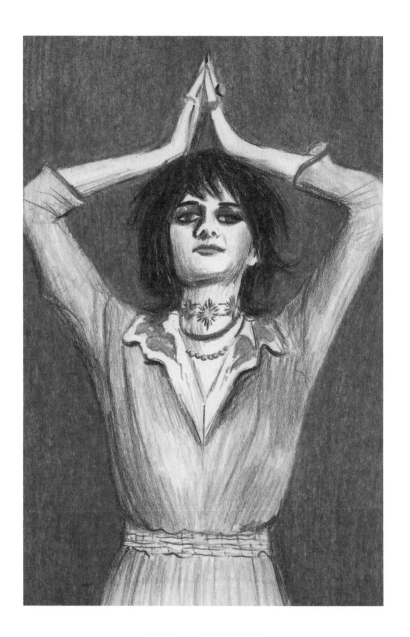

PLATE NO. 9 * JANE ORMSBY-GORE

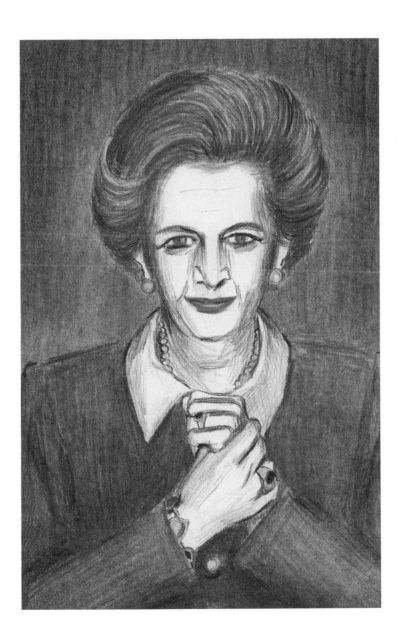

PLATE NO. 10 * MARGARET THATCHER

Ferragamo court shoes with one-inch heels (said shoes enjoyed a kind of Chungian [Alexa] satirical makeover 30 years later).

The lady herself wore her tailoring and unmistakable champagne-coloured, bouffant hairdo like armour (she also co-reigned over the birth of a very important tribe in the Eighties – the Sloanes; see the Tribes of Britannia chapter).

For Mrs – now Baroness T – to be casually dressed was to wear her jacket slung round her shoulders while pouring tea for Denis or sipping scotch on the sofa with members of her dishy all-male, elegantly suited cabinet, in particular Cecil Parkinson and Michael Heseltine.

Mrs T was never without her Ferragamo handbag, used to clobber the disobedient ranks. The handbag became a symbol of political authority. 'Have you been handbagged?' became a euphemism for 'Have you been sacked?' Thatcherism might be a dirty word (and an ideology) but Mrs T's no-nonsense fashion sense has become synonymous with Eighties Britannia. It is recognised as a historical style with a timeless appeal.

KATE MOSS — Whatever happened to that 14-year-old with freckles and wonky teeth who pioneered spaghetti straps and a skewed kind of undone beauty? You only have to hear her cackle to know she's still with us, which is reassuring given her rise to style icon and business tycoon.

Where Kate-the-girl-next-door meets Kate-the-image is in the vintage dresses, the diamonds with denim, the hooded eyes and the ratty blonde hair. Her girlishness hides a steely core, which accounts for her professionalism and longevity. A notorious good-time girl, she's completely inclusive, constantly recruiting new members to her clan (as long as you can keep up). A social chameleon, she plays common-as-muck from Croydon one minute

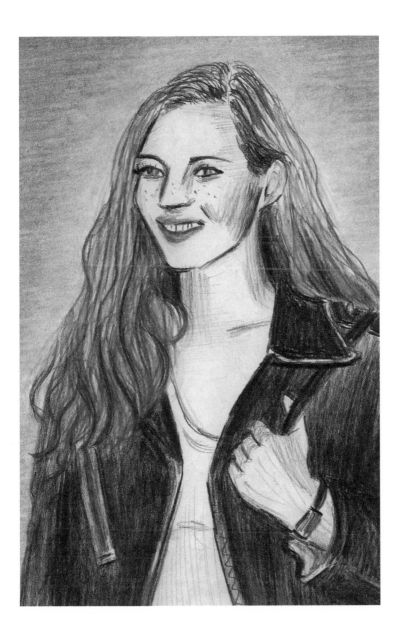

PLATE NO. II • KATE MOSS

and Lady Muck of Gloucestershire the next, but she really doesn't give a crap about social status – why should she, she's Kate, she just enjoys being the character whether it's wellies and waistcoats, jumping out of a chopper in the middle of a field to have a wee, or being the most beautiful vision of glamorous perfection with a glint of mischief in her eye in a gold turban at the Met ball. The thing about Kate is she is genuinely charismatic. She lives the rock and roll dream – once professing to drinking Keith Richards under the table – but is kind, without an ounce of snobbery attached to her. To know her is to be utterly entranced by her.

Fashion calls for reinvention. Kate's look has evolved over the decades, ultimately ending in the selfless gesture of giving it over to her legions of disciples in easy to swallow, not too pricy versions of her wardrobe by way of Kate Moss for Topshop and immediately blurring the lines between high street and fashion.

Despite her fame, her extraordinary otherness, she remains the Artful Dodger. If you have any further doubt just think back to those Kate and Johnny Depp days, Kate in a white T-shirt, no bra and a leather jacket, or that punky, cute little headshot that David Sims took, defining a moment in fashion that is still poignant today as something that changed perceptions of what beauty could be.

HELENA BONHAM CARTER —

I'm in the stocks perpetually in the UK. They say, 'What is she wearing now? How dare she?' Like, criminal acts ... I have a responsibility now to dress badly so it's kind of liberating.

HELENA BONHAM CARTER

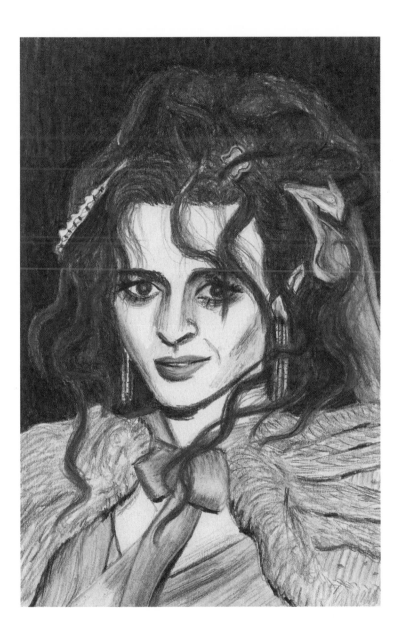

PLATE NO. 12 ∗ HELENA BONHAM CARTER

This bird deserves her place on the list of the most stylish British birds for her sheer contrariness and ongoing disobedience to the dictates of fashion. She is the kind of unique British bird that manages the heroic feat of never abandoning the principles of the first stage of the seven ages. She wears fairy-tale dresses (whether dark and Gothic or innocent and frilly) with utter defiance – Westwood ball dresses day in, week out and always with a pair of stripy socks and multiple hair accessories, naturally fitting right in with her husband Tim Burton's flights of fancy. She can be a dishevelled schoolgirl in ties and Victorian boots one day and a quintessential English bag lady with a madcap ponytail the next. She loves a good vintage satin slip but wears it like she really has just got out of bed – she looks, admirably, like she can't resist throwing herself heartily at every village hall jumble sale going. She once created a line of clothes called 'pantaloonies' that consisted of bloomers and Victorian camisoles, with not a care for market research and not a thought for the demand for such niche attire.

Her family background is impeccably eccentric and eclectic, numbering a prime minister (Asquith), Ian Fleming and Florence Nightingale as relations – which must provide some of the confidence required to be a brilliantly batty British bird.

She is also a brilliant actress – Marla Singer in *Fight Club* is one of my all-time favourite characters – and she consistently chooses roles that are iconic beacons of English womanhood: the Red Queen, Enid Blyton, Mrs Lovett and Lucy Honeychurch, to name but a few of the magic sprinkles she has cast on to our imaginations.

TOP TEN
BRITISH BIRDS

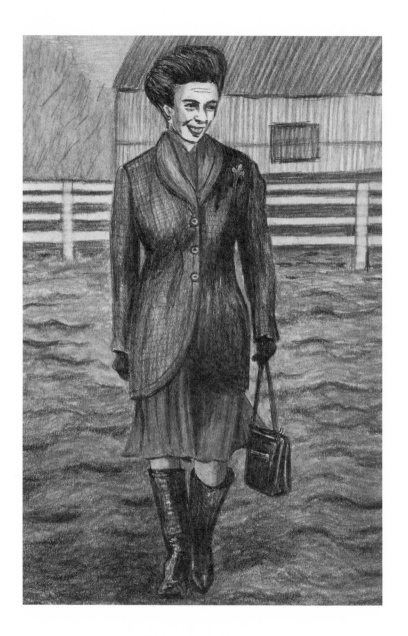

PLATE NO. 13 • PRINCESS ANNE

PRINCESS ANNE (1950−)

SPECIES — ROYAL

SUBSPECIES — ZARA PHILLIPS

HABITAT — BADMINTON HORSE TRIALS

BEHAVIOUR — OLYMPIC HORSEWOMAN, RECKLESS DRIVER,
CHARITY WORKER

I've had many a heated debate about this one, holding up the writing process quite considerably. Most of my friends and cohorts think the particularly rebellious and wild Princess Margaret should take Princess Anne's place but I stand by my decision to go with Anne. Her mum, the Queen, gets a coveted runner-up rosette and her aunty Margaret probably would do too if that didn't make me look like a scary royalist. But Anne is the one that I have looked to in my many spates of waning inspiration.

Anne is the very cool, androgynous, horsey dude who looked killer in a pair of jodhpurs, and whose extraordinary up-do (I think the technical term is 'the onion') has become part of the Royal Family's mythology and the guardian spirit of a kind of messed-up ponytail of which I am an extreme loyalist. Princess Anne has followed in her mother's footsteps by hanging on to her innate sense of style – namely jodhpurs

unless harangued into wearing something else by family commitments – e.g. royal weddings. But she always manages to keep to the very English rule of looking slightly unkempt in everything.

Like most of my birds, she is so much more than style over content. This particular bird rode in the Olympics, which in itself takes guts and attitude, and it's this passion that informs her style. Even when she's in formal attire she looks like she should be on a horse and you get the feeling she'd rather be living in a horse box than a palace. Another good reason for inclusion is her penchant for androgynous military dressing – who doesn't love a good military jacket over another pastel suit/hat combination, or maybe an oversized blazer, a headscarf, upwards-pointing shirt collar, or a sensible-heeled loafer. Princess Margaret may have had a great line in chiffon and tiaras but I feel my case for Anne is a worthy one.

POLY STYRENE (1957-)

SPECIES — POST-PUNK SCREAMER

SUBSPECIES — LILY ALLEN

HABITAT — THE MAN IN THE MOON PUB IN CAMDEN,
CBGB'S IN NEW YORK

BEHAVIOUR — POLEMIC SINGING, SHOUTING

Poly has been hailed as the least conventional front person in rock history and the archetype for the modern-day feminist Punk. Talented, clever, open-hearted, open-minded and sassy, she stood out thanks to her individualism. She didn't fit with Punk or anything around her; she was just a girl in braces screaming about stuff that was very before her time: the garishness of consumer culture.

When the rest of Punk was wearing leather trousers and ripped T-shirts, Poly was wearing red roses and Day-Glo scarves in her hair, brightly coloured, ill-fitting, frumpy suits, leather shift dresses, white ankle socks, kitten heels and soldier hats. She once said in an interview, 'everyone should wear what they want to wear and not have to go to particular shops, that's not what it's about, it's about self-expression, not imitating other people'. Spoken like a true British bird.

Her look and bearing expressed as much about her polyurethane,

polysexual ideals as her songs did. Her voice was insane and loud – a trained opera singer, she subverted her voice and practically used it as a weapon.

A typical Miss England, at 15 Poly hitched from one music festival to another. Later she found herself in Beaufort Market on the King's Road selling her Day-Glo wares, and was spotted by the manager of the Man in the Moon pub. She was too good a package to miss and so he bought a skinny fluoro tie and gave her a residency in his pub. X-ray Spex was born – producing one iconic album with a cover that has been the longest standing resident on the Luella mood board. X-ray Spex played at CBGB's in New York to a crowd that included Blondie, Keith Moon and Richard Hell (who offered himself up as boyfriend material – she didn't take him up on it). Then X-ray Spex imploded, as quick to leave as to arrive. Poly obviously just had better things to do.

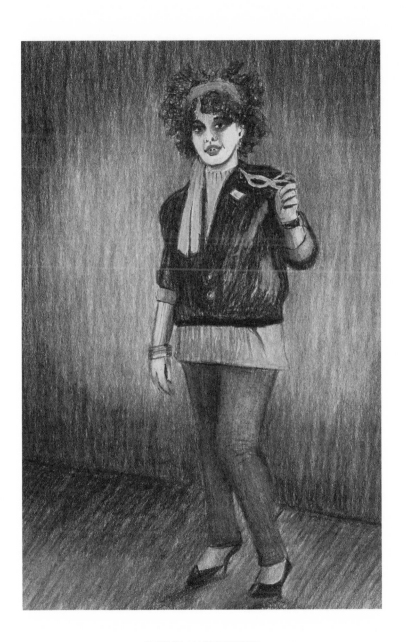

PLATE NO. 14 * POLY STYRENE

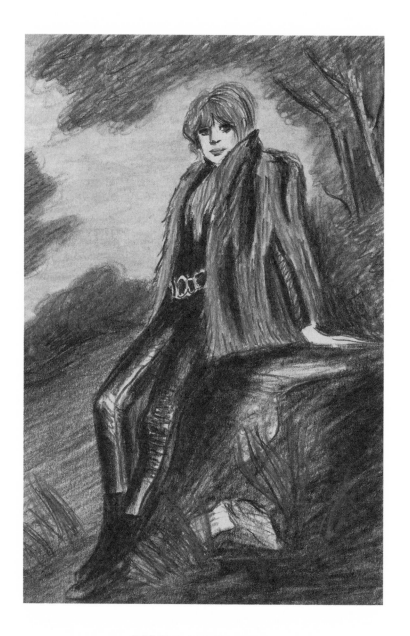

PLATE NO. 15 * MARIANNE FAITHFULL

MARIANNE FAITHFULL (1946–)

SPECIES — MUSE, SONGWRITER

SUBSPECIES — KATE MOSS

HABITAT — CHELSEA, RURAL IRELAND

BEHAVIOUR — EXPERIENCED

No Sixties singer lost her innocence with as much elegance and determination as Marianne Faithfull. Faithfull defined blonde ambition and vulnerability with an angelic convent schoolgirl voice. Lovingly known in the Sixties as 'the angel with big tits', my favourite picture of her is from behind, her blonde hair tied back with a perfectly prim ribbon bow and a pair of Mary Jane's on her feet.

Then came drug addiction, a life shattered, and in 1979 she used her anger in a time of Punk to write her comeback album *Broken English*, sung in a husky, world-weary smoker's cough of a voice. She once owned a pure voice but with the excess it got ravaged and she has said that she now has the voice she deserves.

Faithfull is a progressive soul – saying the woman is experienced is to do her an injustice, although she is another exemplary example of the inimitable English granny, a non-judgemental and wild wise woman. She has been vilified for the things men are revered for, and now when men in music are adored till a ripe old age she is doing the same thing. Her journey, through innocence and playing an intellectual muse (she was the only one on the Rolling Stones tour bus to read books and has used literary references a-plenty in her music), to full-time junkie and actress, to a breast cancer survivor and songwriter, collaborating with the likes of Nick Cave, PJ Harvey and Jarvis Cocker, has been a truly colourful one and she has used all the experience and emotion to make inspiring new music. 'Regret is pointless' seems to be her mantra. She has lived with the tag of Mick Jagger's ex for almost half a century but she is so much more than this now that she's living the bohemian dream in rural Ireland. At a pensionable age, without having been nipped, tucked or Botoxed, she looks enviably good in black leather trousers and a white shirt, with a cigarette still burning on.

MELANIE WARD

SPECIES — STYLIST, DESIGNER

SUBSPECIES — PHOEBE PHILO

HABITAT — NEW YORK AND LONDON

BEHAVIOUR — MILITANT PURVEYOR OF ENGLISH GRUNGE
AND MINIMALISM

> From my childhood through my Grunge years, and even into the whole minimalism thing, I had a certain irreverence towards clothing. I'm not afraid to cut it.
>
> MELANIE WARD

Customising clothes by cutting them up is a Great British habit and Miss Ward is the pioneering force in this particular kind of customisation. It's the wayward cousin of the anarchic precision pattern cutting of our British male designers and is both classical and Punk – a perfect combination. Melanie's genius – when confronted with a piece of clothing, be it a T-shirt, a pair of jeans or a piece of expensive designer clobber – is to make a cut which cheekily tweaks the proportions.

Melanie's most famous cutting moment was when she sliced the top off a pair of Calvin Klein jeans for an iconic mid-Nineties advertising campaign. She also sanded the legs to make them look distressed. That saw the biggest set of lightbulbs for a generation form above the heads of jeans wearers and jeans companies – many millions were made with distressed denim, but Melanie did it first (and it never again looked quite as cool as that first moment). Aside from being impressed by that, pawing over her shoots in *The Face* was also formative stuff for me.

Melanie was Helmut Lang's right-hand woman – his creative director in the Nineties – and had a huge impact on the direction of the collections. She was an essential part of the design process, her irreverence being clear throughout. When the Helmut Lang paint-splattered jeans first appeared I laughed – and then became one of the army of folk walking around looking like painters and decorators. Like the nylon, winged top that seemed to float down the runway, the clothes had a kind of conceptual wit and defined a moment beautifully.

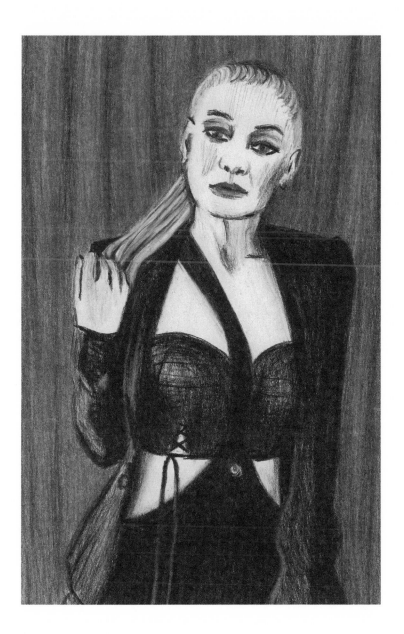

PLATE NO. 16 * MELANIE WARD

Throughout her career Melanie has consistently served up classic sexiness and femininity mixed with militant and cheeky conceptualism, accompanied by a hefty dose of rebellion and some gentle insolence. Does the fact that she was educated by nuns have anything to do with it? Melanie's is a kind of pared-down style. She is a determined perfectionist and a defiant minimalist but a believable one. She must have had a huge effect on the brilliant designs of another clever British bird, Phoebe Philo, who is now seducing the world with her own radical but wearable classicism.

Melanie was, after all, possibly the first to wear a man's dinner jacket to a party as a dress. The French might lay claim to having worn a dinner jacket dress to a party, but you can bet that dinner jacket was cut to perfectly fit the woman's form – Melanie just simply, and brilliantly, borrowed a jacket. Yes, The Ward can lay claim to furthering the cause of those of us who like to steal clothes from our boyfriends too.

We have many incredibly clever stylists in England – the girls and boys who have a very special eye for a twist that can sum up an image or a character succinctly, and who know how to put a good look together to surprise or clarify or subvert, and we all know which nation is best at that. There are many stylists who deserve more than a mention in this list but none has had such an effect on me personally as Melanie. It was without doubt her interpretation of Grunge (along with David Sims) that made it such a stylish and radical movement.

KATE BUSH (1958–)

SPECIES — SINGER, SONGWRITER, DANCER,
CHOREOGRAPHER, PRODUCER, SET DESIGNER,
COSTUME DESIGNER, MIME ARTIST

SUBSPECIES — P J HARVEY

HABITAT — COUNTRYSIDE

BEHAVIOUR — DRAMA, RUNNING UP HILLS IN WALES

Let me take you to a time of sweet personal nostalgia. Me, aged seven, sitting on the sheepskin-rugged floor in front of my mum who was making tiny plaits in my freshly washed hair. This would usually happen the night before a special occasion and she would do hers too. The next morning we would wake up, take out the plaits and become living odes to Kate Bush, albeit blonde versions. It is one of my favourite memories of the Seventies. I was very young when Kate Bush was at her arm-flailing peak. But those overtheatrical gestures would manifest themselves in my mother like a modern dance unfolding in our tiny terrace house in Stratford-upon-Avon.

There is no other British bird quite as exotic as Kate Bush (albeit in a very cold, wet, English landscape), no bird with quite so many feathers, so colourful a plumage and such a mesmerising sound.

Her brand of eccentric pagan abandon was English sensuality at its very best. Everyone – man, woman, beast – was turned on by Kate Bush, who, in turn, said she was genuinely unaware of her sexual allure and much more concerned with her artistic endeavours (boyfriends are for mere mortals). She was just experimenting with all of those strange extrovert pastimes that are oh-so-natural to a very typical type of free-spirited English woman – most of whom end up teaching drama or sculpture to embarrassed teenagers and having the odd affair with the more mature ones. I had one (a teacher, not an affair), and her name was Stella. School wasn't so inspiring for Ms Bush and she said that it inhibited her, which stands to reason; what school could cater for such an individual? She wrote 'The Man with the Child in His Eyes' when she was thirteen.

Kate was certainly ethereal, and nothing if not surreal, dabbling in the arts of circus, dance, mime (given rock and roll status by David Bowie), folk, poetry, literature, performance art, sculpture and the violin – but she did it all with a sense of darkness. She came out of Punk and everything she did was anarchic and a lot of her music was inspired by personal terrors and nightmares. We can all be wanton fairies running up hills, but a typical Miss England will invariably do it with a slightly darker subtext. Her uniform consisted of leotards, scarves, footless tights, sandals or bare feet, ballet tutus (worn with a dunce's cone hat), velvet, mohair, a healthy dose of Bill Gibb, loads of make-up and on occasion animal costumes – apart from Kurt Cobain I can't think of anyone else who can make animal costumes look meaningful. She designed all her costumes, as well as her sets and videos and anything else she could think of. She is the ultimate inspiration for just doing what the hell you want without restriction. You want to make a dress – you make it; you want to design sets – do it; you want to dance – dance. Degrees are a modern disease, creativity just *is*.

Oh and one other rather outthere Bushism (and here's another pattern among my group of distinguished British birds: along with self-destruction she loved her cats) is this. Her cats were called Pywacket and Zoodle. Enough said.

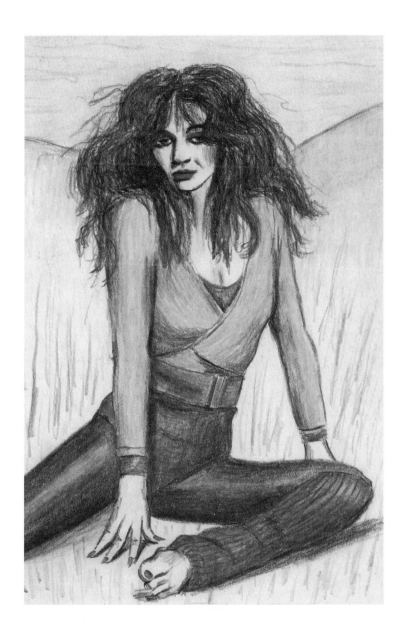

PLATE NO. 17 • KATE BUSH

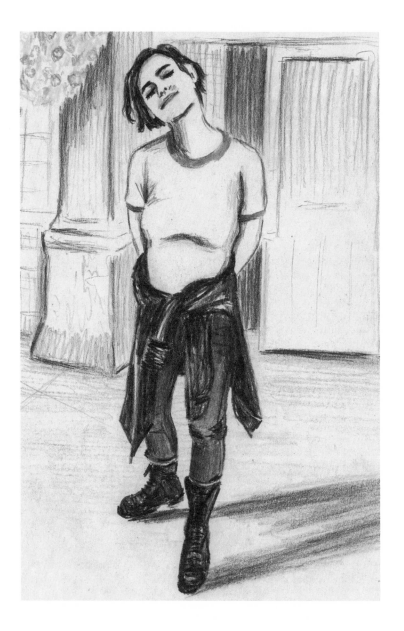

PLATE NO. 18 * JUSTINE FRISCHMANN

JUSTINE FRISCHMANN (1969–)

SPECIES — MUSICIAN, TRAINED IN ARCHITECTURE

SUBSPECIES — M.I.A.

HABITAT — NOTTING HILL, CAMDEN

BEHAVIOUR — INTELLECTUAL POP STAR

Tall, tomboyish, elegant and fiercely clever, Justine was, along with her band mates – Donna Matthews and Annie Holland – the strident cool girl in the early Nineties Britpop phenomenon. These were girls who looked like beautiful boys. Justine never veered from her personal style manifesto of jeans, Dr Martens and baggy T-shirts, which hung over her legendary boobs – knackered T-shirts certainly look their best with a good pair of boobs underneath. It seemed like every boy in a band at that time fancied Justine, which for the rest of us meant it was now firmly okay to look scruffy, wear jeans, be clever and still find a mate.

She was no groupie though. With Elastica she had a hugely successful band of her own achieving more success in the United States than any of her Britpop peers. One of my all-time personal favourites: best name, best lyrics, best attitude – oh Elastica, how I miss thee. Post-Elastica she went on to front a

programme about her other passion – architecture.

She was influenced by The Pixies, The Clash and The Stranglers, and when she strapped on a guitar and sang sixty-second, honest, funny, tough love songs about Vaseline from behind a floppy black fringe it inspired a generation of boyish young girls to step up. 'Car Song' had particular meaning for me and my then flat mate, Katie Grand. It gave our Ford Fiesta a kind of iconic new lease of life, even when it wouldn't start. I remember embroidering the lyrics on a denim jacket in a rather teenage fan moment.

The first thing you notice about Justine, after her imposing dark coolness, is her intelligence. Questioning everything and debating everything.

I had the honour of sharing a house with Justine for a couple of years and was privy to her rather splendid array of vintage T-shirts (long before they became a mass-produced uniform for every girl under 30).

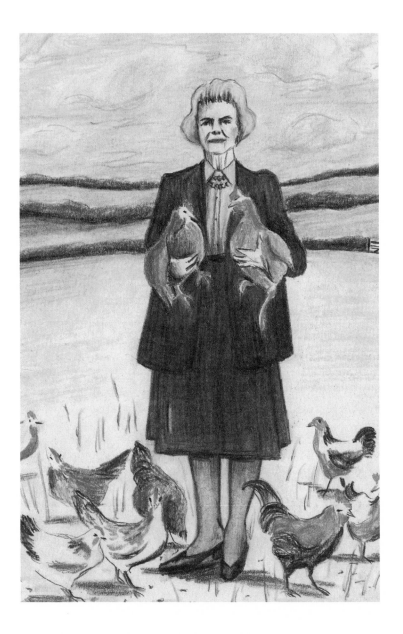

PLATE NO. 19 * THE DUCHESS OF DEVONSHIRE

THE DUCHESS OF
DEVONSHIRE (1920-)

SPECIES — DOWAGER DUCHESS, AUTHOR OF *COUNTING MY
CHICKENS AND OTHER HOME THOUGHTS*

SUBSPECIES — STELLA TENNANT (HER GRANDDAUGHTER)

HABITAT — CHATSWORTH

BEHAVIOUR — PRACTICAL

> I buy most of my clothes at agricultural shows, and good stout things they are. After agricultural shows, Marks & Spencer is the place to go shopping, and then Paris. Nothing in between seems to be much good.
>
> THE DUCHESS OF
> DEVONSHIRE

The youngest of the six Mitford sisters, the Duchess of Devonshire epitomises tweedy, practical, aloof country elegance with wit and a certain kind of privileged nod to self-deprecation. She personifies post-War perfection: the perfectly coiffed hair, the strands of pearls, and the belief in good quality cashmere and a well-made Italian shoe. It is a kind of perfection that has both gone out of fashion and inspired a Miss England like me to revere it and take a sardonic scissor to it. Indeed, her

own blood (Stella Tennant) did just this, combining impeccable breeding with a commendable understanding of the values of Grunge. I'm sure her grandmother dotingly approved – in other words, she got it.

Her generation insisted on good manners, ramrod posture and daily letter writing. The letters to her sisters, Birdie, Cord, Woman, Decca and The Old French Lady are full of arch, upper-class humour and gossip – posh, well-written *Heat*. Everyone is either in fits of gloom or terrific spirits and Nancy's weakness for Christian Dior doesn't go unnoticed. The Duchess has been known to feed the chickens in Jean Patou, Balmain and Chanel couture evening gowns – and wellies. She still wears a Givenchy dress purchased in 1958: like I said, always utterly practical in the face of sheer decadence.

In 1950 her husband, Andrew,

inherited the title Duke of Devonshire and Chatsworth – the Devonshire family estate – and she forsook city life for country pursuits. Loyal patrons of Lucian Freud (they became friends in the Forties), the Duke and Duchess owned fourteen of his paintings. She was painted by Lucian Freud (Lu) in 1961; her (late) husband, the Duke, shared a love of horses and racing with Freud and bought a portrait of a rear view of a horse for the Duchess, which was unveiled at a ceremony at Chatsworth in 2004.

Famed for her love of animals – in particular chickens, hence her nickname Hen – she merrily compares chickens to ladies who shop.

DAME VIVIENNE WESTWOOD (1941–)

SPECIES — FASHION DESIGNER

SUBSPECIES — NONE

HABITAT — KING'S ROAD, LONDON

BEHAVIOUR — CONTRARY

> For me Mrs Thatcher has always been one of the world's best-dressed people. Her politics were appalling but her look gave her incredible presence.
>
> DAME VIVIENNE WESTWOOD

There are two queens of England. There's the Establishment one who deals with all the formal stuff, like the Trooping of the Colour and taking tea with the prime minister and random global dignitaries (that one wears lemon), and then there's Queen Viv, our other beloved sovereign, who takes care of the country's left side of the brain, its image as a creative and vibrant force in the world. Queen Viv's empire has been going strong for thirty years, consistently proving our great nation to be the superior creative power it is, while commenting (in a particularly soft, dry, Alan Bennett-esque voice) on every part of English history and social hierarchy, serving as a reminder that when it comes to style, wit, tradition and rebellion we control the entire world.

Westwood is the perennial nonconformist; she has been laughed at, ridiculed, reviled for her designs and her views, until, one day, the country finally came round to her way of thinking. Nowadays she is loved, applauded and honoured by the other queen, and by the country. Although I sometimes, even now, detect a subtle hint of condescension in her new tag of eccentric national treasure. Her art has changed attitudes, inspired youth movements (Punk, New Romantics) and provoked political thinking. She is our greatest, cleverest, wittiest commentator on the British psyche and she has never compromised her ideas, even when they have set her against the popular establishment, be it fashion or otherwise. She always seems slightly indifferent to praise, almost smirking at the people who lavish it on her.

Now a silver-horned flame-haired granny, Westwood has turned anti-fashion into an identifiably English brand renowned for its couture quality, tailoring and historicism. By 1971, Westwood, with her scruffy, bleached hair, manifested the country's youthful anger and unrest by selling customised T-shirts, which she ripped, knotted and emblazoned with 'Fuck', 'Rock' and 'Perve', in her first King's Road boutique Let It Rock – it was almost playschool in its brilliantly anarchistic simplicity.

Thus the politicisation of clothing was born, paving the way for Punk. As the co-owner of the renamed SEX with former husband Malcolm McLaren, she reinvented fetish-wear as a street style. In the Eighties Westwood turned a 500-year-old shirt pattern into her inspiration for the Pirate collection. The Pirate collection, and her Punk collections, and Witches collections, were unisex, and the ideas behind them are still prevalent now – who hasn't visited Steven at Rellik and pleaded with him to part with those really iconic pieces? Then came a fascination with old world decadence and the French Royal Court, resulting in collections that some viewed as crazy fancy dress with their exag-

gerated sleeves and corsetry, but they were always before their time.

Westwood's trick has been to subvert traditional English style (military, equestrian, ballroom) with intelligence and wit. She plays on the notion of Britishness and parodies traditional upper-class attire, using dramatic cuts to undermine perceptions of scale. Her key is to make it wearable. She has championed traditional fabrics, such as Harris Tweed, lambswool, tartan and velvet (this is where Teddy Boys and Kensington schoolchildren meet) and turned the meanings of the centuries, and decades, into a movable feast. 'I would describe it as a nostalgia for the future,' she has said.

The thing with Westwood the designer is that she can do everything. She is a master craftswoman, an ironist, an intellectual commentator. She can do modern, classical, theatrical; she is a traditionalist, an activist and a rebel. And she has a sharp, didactic sense of humour and she's as nutty as a fruitcake. There is no other designer who embodies all these traits – most are revered for having just one or two of these qualities.

Her 1989 *Tatler* cover, dressed up as Mrs T, became a defining Eighties image.

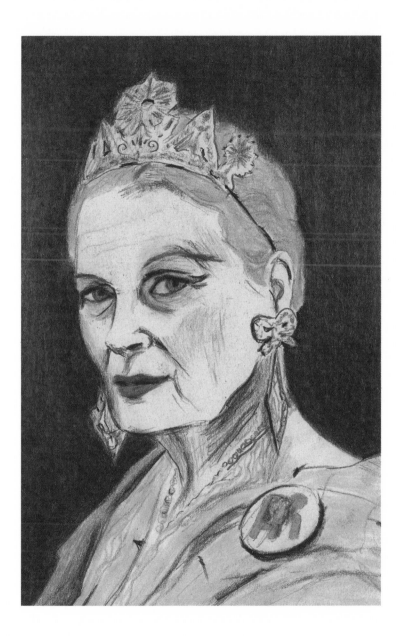

PLATE NO. 20 ✦ DAME VIVIENNE WESTWOOD

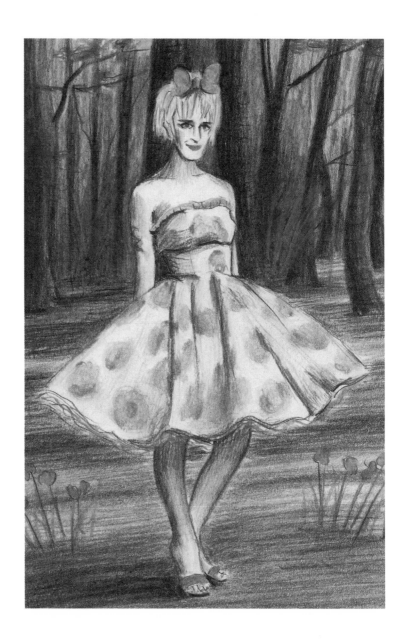

PLATE NO. 21 • PAULA YATES

PAULA YATES (1959–2000)

SPECIES — GROUPIE, AUTHOR, MODEL, MUM, TV PRESENTER

SUBSPECIES — PIXIE, PEACHES

HABITAT — CONDUCTING INTERVIEWS
WITH ROCK STARS IN BED

BEHAVIOUR — 'I'M WITH THE BAND'

As a Boomtown Rats groupie, 17-year-old Paula, a giggly but ultimately razor sharp peroxide blonde, was known as 'The Limpet'. She was the original wild child. Then she married Bob (Geldof) and the fantasy princess who could flirt for Britain (and made a brilliant career out of it) became a witty media-babe. Paula's career spanned television presenting, magazine journalism and penning best-selling books on babies, on sex ('Can I get pregnant with my pants on?'), on blondes and on rock stars in their underpants. For girls growing up in the Eighties, long before the rise of the supermodel, there was Paula, the nation's naughty big sister. Between 1982 and 1987 Friday afternoons were devoted to watching Paula making trouble on *The Tube*, using whiny flirtation to convince Sting to remove his trousers, which, of course, he did.

A vision of tulle and satin, nautical stripes and red lips, Paula did old-fashioned Hollywood glamour in flouncy Fifties prom dresses, Capri pants and Minnie Mouse bows. She lived out her very own version of *La Dolce Vita*. She traced her passion for Fifties fashions to her father's stash of America's favourite family magazine, the *Saturday Evening Post*. 'The magazines became the foundation of a lifetime's dreams. Here was reality,' she said. She championed Eighties designers Bruce Oldfield and Anthony Price and was married in a scarlet Jasper Conran dress. Her feminine curves were offset with a psychobilly quiff and a green dragon tattoo on her upper arm. This was Paula's paradox: her masculine force and womanly *savoir faire* were hidden behind her cartoonish sex appeal. Paula made being a minx look kind of clever.

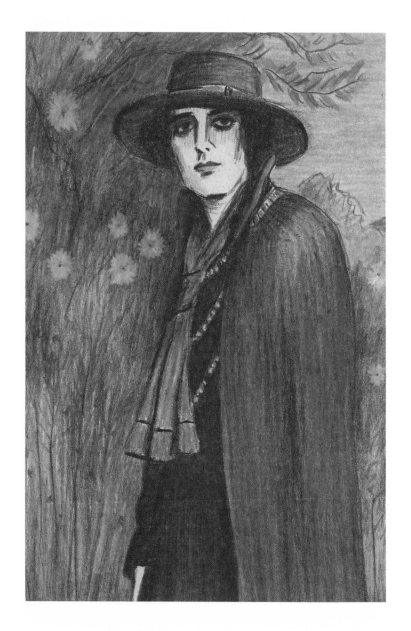

PLATE NO. 22 * VITA SACKVILLE-WEST

VITA SACKVILLE-WEST
(1892–1962)

SPECIES — ARISTOCRATIC POET, NOVELIST, TRAVEL
WRITER, BIOGRAPHER, GARDENER

SUBSPECIES — TILDA SWINTON

HABITAT — SISSINGHURST CASTLE, KENT

BEHAVIOUR — ANDROGYNOUS AND MINIMALIST

Long before boyfriend dressing, there was cross-dressing. In common with Coco Chanel – who in the Twenties borrowed the tweed suits of her paramour the Duke of Westminster – Vita Sackville-West felt at home in men's clothes. Rejecting corsets and the Edwardian taste for fussy ornate blouses with tucks, embroidery, appliqué, lace and pleats, she cut a romantic figure in the fashionable hats of the period, worn with wider brims, which suited her rather male face. She also favoured men's trilbies and Spanish fedoras, an ode to her part-Spanish ancestry. Gamekeeper's breeches were worn with boots laced to the knee; long strings of pearls fell from heavy corduroy jackets tightened with men's leather belts.

Vita's attitude to marriage (her diplomat husband Harold Nicolson referred to her affairs as 'muddles') was as unconventional as her dress sense. In 1918, dressed as a young man in breeches and gaiters, she ran away to Europe with Mrs Violet Trefusis, a novelist. Vita made no secret of her 'duality' (bisexuality). She referred to her masculine side as 'Julian'. According to Virginia Woolf, with whom she had an affair (Vita was the model for *Orlando*), Vita was virginal, savage and patrician. She was a nature-lover known for creating the gardens at Sissinghurst from nothing.

She idealised the role of the female intellectual and the English creative eccentric. She was romantically attached to the countryside and its traditions. Her long poem of 1926 *The Land* gives a portrait of agricultural practices in Kent in particular, England in general.

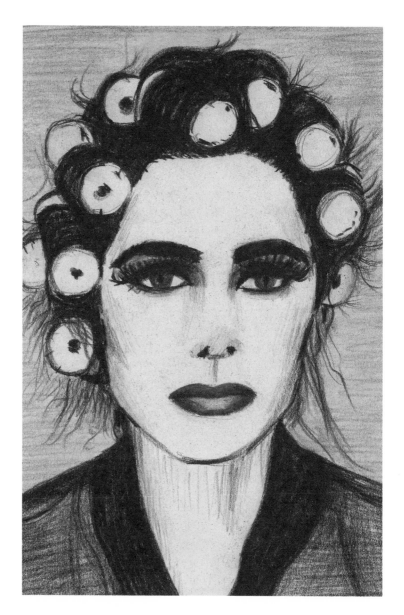

PLATE NO. 23 * PJ HARVEY

PJ HARVEY (1969–)

SPECIES — POST-PUNK BLUES SINGER, SONGWRITER

SUBSPECIES — FLORENCE AND THE MACHINE

HABITAT — DORSET

BEHAVIOUR — A RECLUSIVE EXTROVERT

You can't beat the sight of a girl on stage with the wind in her hair, playing a guitar in a mini and spike heels. I bring you Polly Jane Harvey, unafraid of showing off her pins or expressing her violent emotions. When she first appeared on the scene back in 1991, she was a skinny art school student modestly dressed in leggings and Dr Martens. Catapulted on to the international stage with the massive success of her million-selling albums, she transformed herself into a vamp. Like a scary drag queen, she lost her way in a world of smeared make-up and sequin-covered catsuits. Her need to rage against the world, protesting at being an object of desire while courting popularity in skimpy outfits, was testimony to her twisted sense of beauty, and self.

Then she found herself again. Androgynous, tomboyish, fierce, sexy, defiant, she challenges conventional ideas of beauty with her jolie-laide looks. Her big guitar noise and riffs on love and loss, menstruation, and amputating men's legs have earned her the reputation of sorceress when, in fact, she is a poet with *soul*. These days, like all those West Country Punks, PJ Harvey has matured into an ethereal pale-faced woman with Gothic tendencies. She still churns out abrasive, gut-wrenching songs about betrayal, backed by a bunch of blokes in trilbies, but she does it in floaty black dresses with bare feet and a half-smile. She has mellowed with age – but hasn't given up the fight.

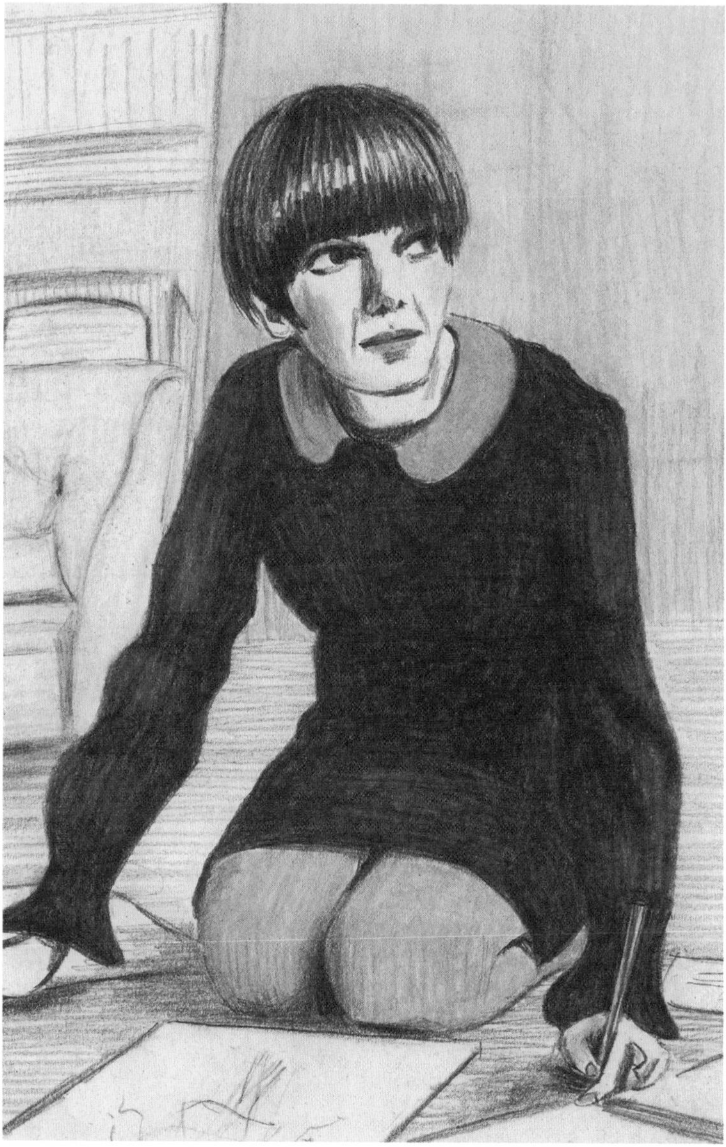

PLATE NO. 24 * MARY QUANT

MARY QUANT (1934–)

SPECIES — FASHION DESIGNER

SUBSPECIES — TOPSHOP

HABITAT — KING'S ROAD, LONDON

BEHAVIOUR — MODERNISER

Miss Mary Quant – how could I have imagined a career in fashion without Mary Quant? She created the miniskirt for heaven's sake. Forgive me – where would Topshop be without her? She also created the idea of Saturday night dressing, making things 'upstairs' that literally came off the machine and into her King's Road shop that day in order to serve her adoring fans' weekend characters.

Whenever I am at a loss I reread her autobiography, which is one of the most inspiring books I have ever read. Quant emerged at the heart of London's Swinging Sixties to save girls from the buttoned-up Fifties; all those bowed dresses and little white gloves. She was the first to design, make and sell miniskirts and tunic dresses from her King's Road boutique Bazaar, which opened in 1955. By the mid-Sixties, Quant had raised hemlines (and shifted social attitudes) eight inches above the knee. Quant represented sex and blissful glorious youth in tandem with the explosion of pop culture.

She created inexpensively made clothing for the new, urban lifestyle. Rather than buying outfits for specific occasions, separates could be purchased in a line called Ginger Group, which 'gives you every season clothes that all go together'. Items included the French cricket skirt, the Miss Muffet dress and the Liberty lawn dress. Later on came the micro-mini and the raincoat. She popularised monochrome at a time when the world was simpler, more black and white, and two-tone was the antidote to the psychedelic hot-pants and ethnic garb for sale at Granny Takes a Trip and at Biba. Her make-up range ('paintbox' make-up, nail-polish colours including white) solved the problem of where to shop for bare essentials and her tights ensured decency when bending over. Quant went on to design for Topshop, which opened in 1964.

LILY ALLEN (1985–)

SPECIES — MOCKNEY SINGER

SUBSPECIES — TBC

HABITAT — MYSPACE, TWITTER

BEHAVIOUR — FRANK

Lily emerged like an exotic bird with her jet-black hair, prom dresses and gobby attitude. Stroppy and opinionated, she is the face of today's twentysomethings who live out their affairs on Facebook, drink too much and manifest all the very worst aspects of Englishness when they're pissed – and when they're online (uninhibited, loutish and generally obnoxious). But all is forgiven because as well as possessing sultry starlet looks and an ability to carry off a Sixties hairdo (the flip, the pixie, the beehive), Lily Allen is funny – she's a tease, and a rather coarse and naive prophet. Her lyrics are an object lesson in how to mix street with sweet. They crackle with bawdy tales of bad sex, celebrity sadness, 'I don't know how I'm meant to feel any more', and political rabble-rousing.

Like a comic book character, Lily flip-flops between being in charge – a grown-up with a TV show and hit albums – and playing the lost little girl. As Cecil Beaton once said of Marilyn Monroe, 'she is an urchin pretending to be grown up'. With success has come grooming; the hair has got glossier, there is that collection of Chanel 2.55 handbags (and a Chanel campaign) and she's learned how to run from the paparazzi in vertiginous heels – while smoking a fag. Placing her in the top ten British birds may be contentious. Although she may not be adept at putting a look together, I find myself loving the crass mistakes, and while she may not be as intellectually sound as some of her contemporaries, her conflict between rebellion and insecurity is undeniably hallmark British. She's got that English girl nous, and what your teacher would call filthy language, thereby ensuring her place amongst the ranks of British birds.

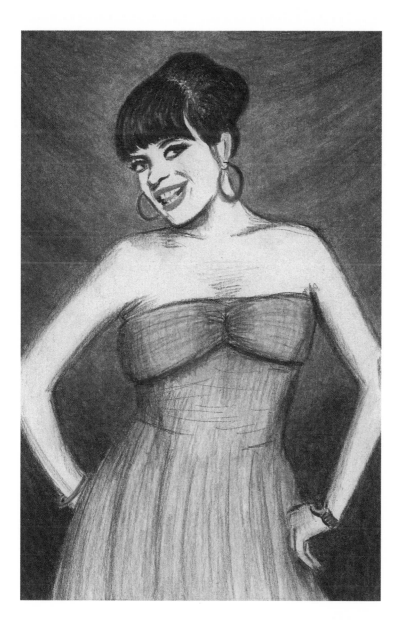

PLATE NO. 25 ● LILY ALLEN

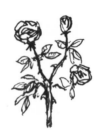

LOVE, SEX
& TOMBOYS

A TALE OF TWO KNICKERS — An admission: when it comes to sex, the more prudish, comfortable-shoe side of the British bird's nest is where I like to nestle. Like many British birds I can do it – and enjoy it – but talking about it tends to bring on some umbrage. I may prefer my hair to look like I've just done it, but I don't dress in a way that suggests I'm trying to attract anyone solely for the purpose of it.

I live in Cornwall now – not that that's got anything to do with all this – but on my fortnightly visits to London I now find myself rather scandalised by the unexpected wares to be found in the capital's most revered underwear shops. At Agent Provocateur (the pioneer of twenty-first-century British knicker establishments) and Coco de Mer (the more probing, out-there younger sister of AP), ornate spanking paddles and bejewelled sex toys can be found resting beside the pretty silk and lace smalls (at Coco de Mer an innocuous-looking gold ring can be bought which apparently holds one's fingers in the correct position for perfect masturbation).

I'm all for raffish splendour in knickers – in fact, it seems of fundamental importance considering our love of a tomboyish exterior – and no one would want a Miss England to repress her wildest boudoir desires, however testing to my personal priggish demeanour the requisite accessories might be. But while the frothy balconettes and ranks of leather wrist cuffs reflect something of a typically English attitude to sex – and who wouldn't applaud letting your imagination run riot – the new, calculating brazenness on offer seems to ignore some of the things closest to Miss E's heart: the recklessness of real romance and the true sincerity that makes frosted cynicism melt.

There's plenty to say about love, sex and Miss E – the eternally recurring themes that forever strike a chord with the English girl, and the newly constructed streets she's been invited to tentatively tread down recently – but the best place to begin is with the great Agent Provocateur versus Marks & Spencer debate. This high-street sex war beautifully illustrates two conflicting impulses Miss E is prey to: naughtiness, irreverence and adult depravity versus stuff-and-nonsense familiarity and practicality. While Joe Corre, Agent Provocateur's co-founder, is the son of Malcolm McLaren and Vivienne Westwood, it's no coincidence that Margaret Thatcher confessed to buying her underwear at Marks & Spencer. AP versus M&S: this is a tale of two knickers, a classic English fable.

Marks & Sparks is an English institution, a consumerist homage to middle England, and a one-stop shop for the middle classes to hide in, wallow in and buy good value cashmere sweaters, carefully counted daffodils and ready-chopped vegetables. It's the twinset of the high street, promising to bring Peter Jones values to those dwelling outside Chelsea. Marks & Spencer is a bit frumpy and safe but in rather a lovely way. The powers that be in the boardroom try to modernise it but nothing really changes, it just coats whoever is trying, yet again, to make it cool with its unchanging and comfortable frumpery. Take new M&S face V. V. Brown, who in her day job sings Indie, Punky pop, and now looks extremely normal – beautiful but comfy. (Like oil, the middle-of-the-road look sticks to anyone who gets too close.)

Frequenting Marks & Spencer is a bit like going back to the bedroom you had as a teenager – it all just looks a bit smaller. One day you think you've outgrown it; feelings akin to Alice in the White Rabbit's house surface. But when you're actually in that space, it feels like you are enveloped in a cuddly, melancholic homesickness. The underwear department gives me that weird, warm feeling the most. It takes me back to a time when puberty felt like a particularly embarrassing practical joke that everyone was privy to except me, and when Marks & Spencer held out its slightly wrinkly, chubby hand and offered protection in the way of a first bra – a practical little number, nothing alarming and nothing to attract any unnecessary attention to my developing tits. It's soothing to the soul to know that granny pants and training bras still exist; they'll always be there in Marks & Spencer where they embody English frumpery in its most snug form. If my granny didn't still send me a three-pack of white cotton knickers every birthday I would feel just a little out of my comfortable place.

Agent Provocateur, on the other hand, stands for modern Miss E, cool wickedness and oo-er missus glamour, providing the kind of impropriety that the English once secretly, but now more openly, crave. Joe Corre and Serena Rees were the first to make burlesque outfits and spanking paddles seem modern and sophisticated; they were the first to make buying diamante-handled whips to match your suspenders a credible lifestyle choice. The company was founded only in 1994 but now feels like a solid piece of the English cultural landscape. Mrs Beckham famously acquired a plethora of glamorous sex paraphernalia from Agent Provocateur with the same must-have desperation she exercises when buying any of the season's It accessories. Does Agent Provocateur's success mean the English are now willing to be open about sex as long as it has a designer price tag?

With Serena's coy femininity and Joe's innate sense of rebellion and desire to shock, they opened their first shop in Soho on Broadwick Street – a stone's throw from haunts like the Raymond Revue bar (where Joe would later host his burlesque nights). Joe and Serena made sex and being saucy fashionable and created a new kind of underwear that would even seduce the likes of me into being sexy. Just entering their sumptuous changing rooms made you feel special and like you might just pass as an amateur burlesque artiste (lighting has a lot to do with it); not a stripper but a grown-up burlesque artiste, something an M&S changing room was unlikely to bestow. Agent Provocateur is a magical world of possibility – and Serena and Joe even had a clever victory over the forces of frumpery when they entered the enemy's vast cotton-briefed camp by way of a tactical collaboration with Marks & Spencer, turning M&S pilgrims' attention away from their mildly ignorant priorities of comfort and common sense to the delights of a more progressive and ornate pack of three.

Miss E will probably forever feel pulled to the reassurance of Marks & Spencer, then bored by its predictability, then drawn to the thrills of Agent Provocateur, then get a bit unnerved by a telescopic whip and choker set and return to Marks & Spencer where the whole process begins again. There is, though, a new player in the game, to further confuse us. Coco de Mer, opened by Sam Roddick, has gone a step further in the quest to sell grown-up sexual liberation to uptight English folk and the daughters of Sloanes. Coco de Mer's plans are as well thought out as Agent Provocateur's – again combining credibility and luxury – but Coco de Mer wants to push Miss E's boat even further into the uncharted waters of uninhibited adult pleasure.

Where Agent Provocateur is flirty and a bit of Fifties fetishist fun – their windows looking like a cross between a Betty Page bondage photograph and a *Carry On* film – Sam Roddick and Coco de Mer have big ideas to change our approach to sexuality and erotica and to create an alternative to the existing sex industry. Ms Roddick is openly suggesting to a rather bashful Miss E that she gets her deepest, most cloaked fantasies out in the open, something that goes directly against her sometimes timorously puritanical approach to rumpy pumpy – Coco de Mer's shelves boast a quite extraordinary range of gadgets and leatherwork. But Coco de Mer is a high-end sex shop with intellect. Can sex be intellectual? Intelligent, kinky, rebellious high-end sex sounds like something Miss E might be able to get her teeth into, so to speak. Add humour and we'll really be cooking with gas.

There are some very cool values behind Ms Roddick's brand of sex. Her motivation for the business comes out of her passion for activism and education, and there is a proper agenda behind her approach. Like a truly mutinous British bird with a huge and relevant cause behind her, she is trying to change English attitudes towards sex – for her, both frumps and exploiters are all ripe for transformation. This is a big task on Ms Roddick's part but she's not the only one giving Miss E a gentle nudge into the world of erotica.

Look at all those powerful-looking girls on the cover of a recent issue of British fashion magazine *Love*, naked but for some rope and a pair of stilettos. And everywhere, nowadays, our diffident Miss E turns she is confronted by scarcely ambiguous images of sex. Even I found myself at it not so long ago, designing a handbag named Gisele, whose form took on a very traditional look – a sensible, tan, handheld bag in classic calf, but for the strapping around it, the inspiration for which was the strapping one might find in a dominatrix's dungeon. I thought this was very subversive at the time, but really it wasn't so much about emancipation and was, in fact, a typically English, rather childish tease.

So it seems as if the Marks & Spencer view of sex – comfy, wholesome and not to be discussed – has lost ground recently and that the Agent Provocateurs, Coco de Mers and their numerous cheerleaders have the whip hand. And behind all this lie some big arguments about feminism and sexual politics. Miss E, for what it's worth, thinks that a little harnessing of the studded leather variety is fine, if it's done in an intelligent, grown-up and responsible way – but does it really need to be rammed down Miss Prim England's throat as a sign of how sophisticated and strong women are now? Bracing openness and more extreme sex – to say that's what will make every Miss E feel fulfilled – seems to be missing the point, although I concede it must work for some. Does being tied up and spanked really have anything to do with love – dare I sound so sincere – which is always more exciting than sex? On style grounds alone, I can't see any reason for sexuality to always be overt; in the right hands, I still think there's not much sexier, more tantalising and more subversive than a tea dress.

Perhaps things have gone a bit too far lately with all the cupless bras and leather chokers, as it's in balancing the erotic with the frumpy where English girls are most likely to feel on their favourite ground. Crotchless gym slip, anyone?

Even Madonna – who tried to bring erotica up to date in the early Nineties – was eventually drawn to the world of middle England, and the never-to-be-underestimated power of prim. Leaving New York behind her, she went English, bought a pile in the country, took up riding, wore hacking jackets and flat caps, went to the pub, wrote children's books and probably bought her bras at Rigby & Peller, although perhaps not M & S. Even Madonna couldn't resist the seductive charms of stuffy English priggishness – and the dramatic tension between sex and primness that we English do like no others. Powerful stuff.

Right now, as far as underwear and general attitudes towards sex go, there doesn't seem to be much to be found between the two extremes. There's full-on erotica and there's the formal and slightly priggish and frumpy (the exception, perhaps, is the Queen's bra makers Rigby & Peller, who offer a well-fitted mix of frump and properly scaffolded sexiness). Which way to go? As a pretty typical British bird I find my feathers are feeling a touch ruffled by the rush to no-holds-barred (literally) erotica. But Miss Englands tend to know how to mix the best of both worlds, and that's where our salvation lies – selecting from each to emerge in triumph, wit and creativity intact. On our hallowed shores both frumpery and consenting depravity can be celebrated: usually all in a kind of convoluted, snobbish, confusing and underground way as long as the result is personal and original.

O O - ER M I S S U S — The most peculiarly English thing about sex is that for us, it's inextricably bound up (oo-er missus!) with humour. Other nations celebrate their sexuality but we tend to find it all a bit embarrassing, skirt round the issue, and plump for either a polite fumble with the lights out or, fuelled by drugs and alcohol, full-on sexual decadence.

It's usually only with humour that we find ourselves able to talk about sex – and it's not always particularly dazzling humour. I read somewhere that the English man, after sex, will thank his host for having him and the host will thank him for coming – one just can't help it. The comic euphemisms we use when dealing with sex are testimony to our unshakeable shame about the whole thing. Here, showing how juvenile we really are, are just a few of the descriptions we use for that most spiritual and connecting of acts: boff, cop off, get off with, grope, leg over, roger, romp, snog, quickie, ride (spot the equestrian reference), rumpy pumpy and how's-your-father. Women are totty, a penis is a knob, to be attractive is to be tidy and one who is in the mood is known as randy. Did the English ever actually graduate from the sixth-form common room? Put simply, sex makes the English giggle; to say 'making love' tends to make Miss England cringe.

We titter but we rarely flaunt it, as flaunting anything seems to go against the English puritanical streak – it would be like showing off – as does confessing to enjoying it. The Victorians and their sense of shame and embarrassment have a lot to answer for – even if they did provide us with some rather outstanding pieces of high-collared lace. And the Victorians epitomised better than any other generation our still-hypocritical attitudes to sex, considering it an impolite topic for conversation, while Victoria's son Edward VII had an inexhaustible appetite for clandestine depravation and illicit liaisons (somewhere in the region of fifty-five).

Voyeurism is part of the English bag too. The nation will, from a safe distance, while away hours reading the *News of the World*'s documentation of our beloved MPs getting in a pickle with sadomasochism. The British love of a scandal involving power and a good outfit saw Christine Keeler become an icon. The contrary Ms Keeler's style was sophisticated and demure – comprised of pencil skirts and Fifties suits, always accompanied by an immaculate mid-heel and handbag to accessorise her less than immaculate occupation. Her style made the fall of the Macmillan government a much more satisfying fable. (Keeler later went on to feature in a Bryan Ferry video with her accomplice Mandy Rice-Davies.) As far as British sex scandals go, the more degrading and comic the better – Camilla and Charles and their sex tapes, John Major and Edwina Curry (Yes, Yes, Yes, Prime Minister), the sexual conquests of Boris Johnson. We particularly love embarrassing shenanigans involving the upper classes or the powerful – not only can we steal their garb and look better in it, but we can laugh at them for being ridiculous in bed too. Not that our own sexual practices are any more sane.

Behind the frumpery, of course, it's not just politicians and the upper classes who have a taste for decadence. Many of us are frumpish prudes one minute and wild deviants the next. But surely all that binge drinking, binge sex and feeling really bad about it in the morning – for whatever guilt-ridden mixture of the degrading, shameful and forbidden may have taken place – isn't good for us? Maybe Sam Roddick's ideas for intelligent passion, instead of sniggering booze-fuelled juvenility, at least offer an alternative for some bold souls.

MISS E'S NEMESIS — So, Miss England finds herself torn between the cotton safety of Marks & Spencer and the silken adventure of Agent Provocateur, and intrigued by, but probably not quite brave enough to go for, the uncompromising approach of Coco de Mer – although Sam Roddick's thoughts are certainly modern and grown-up and will find increasing favour with plenty. Miss E wants her relationship with sex to be empowering, but doesn't think that involves pretending to be a Californian porn star; she wants sex to be more than a smutty seaside-postcard joke and doesn't believe that scandalous voyeurism is really her look. There is, however, a big new problem that has reared its hair-extensioned head lately.

You know when a Miss E has gone the wrong way – she finds herself aspiring to a glossy, Barbie-doll-like perfection and, sadly, casts away her creativity and individuality. These unwitting victims are often younger Miss Es, who have, bafflingly, got the idea that dressing like a stripper is empowering, and that polishing their sexual allure is the route to a rewarding existence. It goes hand-in-hand with that vacant look of doll-like perfection and believing that simply aiming to become someone's glamorous girlfriend is a credible career choice (if you're going to aspire to be someone's girlfriend, then at least make it a prime minister – great potential for an ironic frump look – rather than a dull footballer). Being glamorous and hanging on to someone's arm is far less of a success than being cool, independent and creative.

Too many young Miss Englands are picking the wrong icons to follow – a clue to the right ones, I believe, is the Birds chapter – the right ones are subversive and original women, like Poly Styrene or Kate Bush. The wrong ones include the recent squadrons of fake-boobed, fake-tanned, fake-haired failed glamour pusses. This isn't just referring to the parody that is Katie Price, but to the likes of Cheryl, Kylie and all those who care more about their gloss than their originality. It's not to them we should look for inspiration, and it isn't to the goody-goody, hyper-conventional, perfect-cup-cake-making domestic goddesses. Neither offers the path to female enlightenment.

Simply to be desired – that's not a high enough aspiration, certainly not in this Miss E's view. Outfits that say little more than 'look at my body' should be outlawed from one's wardrobe. English style has always – from Vita Sackville-West through Vivienne Westwood to Florence Welch – been about expressing one's intelligence, charm and views through one's choice of image. Style can be a clever, succinct way of expressing who you are and who you want to be – and the result might show you to be the complex creature that you are. If what you're saying is just 'be my boyfriend' then you're not saying much. Looking sexy should always come second to looking interesting – to look interesting is to look beautiful. Clothes should be about expressing your feelings – not trying to inspire a certain feeling in men.

That's not how it's done in our green and pleasantly sceptred isle – we are far too rebellious, far too individual in spirit, to settle for such a pitifully mundane approach to dressing.

The Katie Price tendency – though let's be completely clear, no one woman could claim credit for the scale of this – also seems to involve girlhood becoming less imaginative and more pressured. (Surely there should be no pressure in childhood at all?) Sex has become so mainstream that younger and younger girls are aspiring to unrealistic proportions – they are becoming obsessed with looking faultless when they should be experimenting and having fun. As British birds our flaws are our secret weapon. Even the first stage of the seven ages is being infiltrated by highly flammable princess dreams and the desperation to be pretty. Nowadays, a young Miss E is in danger of heading straight from toddler innocence to boyfriend anxiety by the age of five. I still maintain that old Minnie the Minx is the key to banishing the evil Disney princesses.

Miss Englands should be free in toddlerhood and early girlhood to explore their fantastic imaginations. The impish denizens of my playroom are regularly to be found donning whatever outfit turns them into a butterfly, a spaceman, a fox, the Mad Hatter, a sailor, a rabbit, a clown, a fairy or a knight. Bonkers wigs, face paints, bow ties and top hats are what girls (and boys) need to grow their imaginations and see the possibilities in everything – and just to have fun, without any self-consciousness. Now, though, the high street is littered with cheap, nasty products and producing even cheaper values for girls and young women. Style's most evil villain, Primark, was forced to retract a padded bikini top that was being produced for girls as young as seven. How inherently wrong can you get? There is a big distance between the creativity and individuality that every young girl should have and the crap that Primark is trying to sell them.

It's possible to buy T-shirts for a three-year-old saying 'Future Wag'. Tat that makes a young girl into a miniature piece of arm candy, or a sexualised polyester princess, is only going to have dire consequences for a Miss E's self-esteem and her chances of becoming an eccentric of charm and wit. There are too many clothes on the high street that paint the wearer as some corny under-age seductress.

With the arrival of adolescence, Miss Englands have always applied for membership of a tribe, and begun to express all kinds of complicated statements about class, sex, subversion and irony. But mass consumerism and premature body awareness are putting gentle and intelligent self-expression and creativity in jeopardy. I'm not saying that young girls should be hidden under layers of white cotton and an M&S chastity belt – feminism was right to stop sexuality being seen as some hideous secret that should be anguished over until a husband was secured. But why are young girls being encouraged to dress as cheap, naff and nasty seductresses, to be served up in a shower of glitter?

It's one-dimensional and it's horribly brutal because it cuts off the imagination, instead trying to cram everything into a dull search for sexual allure, rather than encouraging girls to explore what beauty really is, to see things with the sideways glance of the witty and intelligent. Happily, my 12-year-old niece thinks Girls Aloud is the spawn of the devil (although I personally like the way Nicola found, late in the day, her true porcelain beauty). She lives on a diet of Florence and the Machine and wears marbled, multi-coloured tights, Dr Martens, hair bows and tulle skirts. I have faith that the next generation will not be fooled. This book is not just nostalgia for the near extinct British bird but a call to arms. Miss E is alive and well and up for a scuffle with her nemesis.

There are others flying the flag for the true spirit of Miss E – creativity, eccentricity and a warped sense of romance. M.I.A., Florence Welch, Natasha Khan of Bat for Lashes, Pixie Geldof, Romy Madley Croft of The XX, Laura Marling and Lily Allen – all are in their own ways fighting and commenting on the pickle Miss E has found herself in of late. The real Miss E and her eternal celebration of everything contrary is way too strong and subversive for the plastic goddesses of reality TV.

I can't help thinking of another heroine here – not an English one but an American one, and a fictional one at that: Enid Coleslaw. As the heroine of *Ghost World* Enid epitomised a potent but innocent sexuality in her Batgirl mask and Dr Martens. She is a beautiful, bored misfit, the kind we have in abundance in small towns around our own nation, and it's these girls who will take up the struggle against the plastic princesses. Enid exemplifies the cool and mysterious girls who play with their image and explore their own ideas of what's sexy and not sexy. The British birds who exemplify this spirit of playfulness and mystery have a fight on their hands. Will they be replaced by plastic pink canaries singing fake birdsong with polyester wings dyed in new improved hyper colour and hyper femininity that can't fly? Never!

ROMANCE — So with sexuality, a Miss England who presents herself as fake and blatant is a sad cardboard cut-out: sad because she's missing out on the creativity, intelligence and fun that accompanies a more complex suggestion of herself. In my book – literally – sexuality means mystery and the convoluted games we play to attract attention, whether it's from the opposite sex or our own. Sexuality is all about suggestion – or lack of it, when appropriate. It's in our dress that we express our ambiguity, our power struggles and our confusion – dress presents the chance to express our rebellion. We offer a glimpse of our real self, but we don't give it all away at once, for a Miss E is naturally self-effacing and fiercely protective of her privacy. To make a contrast: Katie Price trades on her fake curvature and fake glamour, while Kate Moss is a natural beauty first famed for her youth, lack of pumped-up flesh and lack of glamour. But it's Kate Moss, whose mystery and creativity are always at play, who revels in the greater allure.

We Miss Englands are – I'll say it again – complex creatures, our inner traits just as inconsistent as the clothes we choose. We're known for being reserved to the point of being rude and cold, yet underneath a Miss E is likely to hold no regard for rules and conventions. Behind a veil of cool detachment and pose of uptight traditionalism, she's likely to be nurturing the kinkiest, wildest and most subversive of tastes; behind knowing mockery – such as ironically innocent knickers from Stella McCartney – there may hide sexual idiosyncrasies which she won't compromise with anyone. And when the alcohol is flowing, her exterior pose and interior desires will swim in and out of focus, depending on who you are and where you are standing. As a nation, we thrive on inner conflict but I guess that's what makes British romance so interesting and ultimately difficult.

Wit and satire can go too far and become too omnipresent, and I think that may be something that has taken hold recently. These days, in our conceptualist, ironic society, Punk values have seeped into every nook and cranny of our culture, and this itself can turn into something bland. While we pick our looks from a range of tribes and heritages – mixing and matching to our heart's content – revealing something of who you really are, with no irony, can be forgotten. Our insatiable appetite for wit and satire can make it nigh on impossible to have a loving relationship (though, of course, all of this makes us droolingly tempting and intimidating to men the world over). Irony – and bravado – is our English way of hiding our awkwardness. But with the detachment of irony, even love – the most sincere thing there is – can often be seen as something a bit naff and corny and generally ripe for a good lampooning.

I think that's where I will wrap this up – with an invitation to remember and include the properly Romantic, with all the rush-of-blood sincerity and true passion that it embodies. I don't mean the Barbara Cartland-type of satin-bodice-popping-in-the-conservatory romantic, but Romantic with a capital R, like the Romantic poets, who sewed their fast-beating hearts to their voluminous white cotton sleeves, and the distinguished lineage that followed. Romance and its flamboyance are what we do best – look at Byron, Coleridge, Wordsworth, Shelley, Keats, Vita Sackville-West, Edith Sitwell, Iris Murdoch, Oscar Wilde, David Bowie, Morrissey, Ian Curtis, Kirsty MacColl, Kate Bush and PJ Harvey.

I think it's the dash of intelligent, witty, do-or-die Romanticism that I find missing from the comfort zone of Marks & Spencer, the saucily nudging shelves of Agent Provocateur and the more effortful and demanding wares of Coco de Mer. I would like to think that underneath the more famous English dens of iniquity that serve the rock and roll elite, usually residing in Soho, London, even further underground reside illicit dens of English romance – foppish poets and people of sincerity, writing and reciting Romantic prose, drinking tea through the night, wearing bloomers, hidden from the eyes of the Punk ironists. The darker side of Romanticism – the tumble to personal destruction, anguish and overindulgence – might be less welcome, but it is fundamental to the art of being English too.

Our more practical side may be in conflict with Romanticism, but romance is our principal desire. How could it ever be anything else? Wordsworth wrote passionately about the value of intuition over reason, though both are crucial to the British bird, who balances both in her choice of outfits, and her choice of lover. But in a fight, intuition would win Miss E's heart every time.

ANDROGYNY'S PROGENY — 'A bob, a pair of earrings and a leather handbag – it was basically love at first sight.' This was Justine Frischmann's heartfelt quip on first seeing the ethereal-looking, fine-featured Brett Anderson – shortly to become her boyfriend – flailing foppishly towards her. It's a very English vision – Mills & Boon in dirty jeans. It's all the more authentic, and romantic, for not involving any Jane Austen, unrealistic, empire-lined, husband-obsessed stuff: the costume dramatics here only mean drainpipes and shrunken blazers. This is the real deal: the story of a boy and a girl with a similar taste for a lean boyish body shape – and long fringes to cover their shared exhibitionist introversion. Such a couple are likely to be English.

One can spot them everywhere, knowingly gorgeous twins on love's young parade – same jeans, shoes, hair, accessories, walking arm in arm in narcissistic homage to each other. Shoreditch is undoubtedly the best place to go spotting them, where fun and games can be had unearthing aesthetically delightful pairs. But increasingly you will find such couples and general gender blurring in small provincial towns around the country. We have our very own progeny of androgyny in Wadebridge – my local town – where Indie Emo teenagers with indistinguishable two-tone hairdos can be found snogging outside the Co-op, and long-haired, blonde surf couples, all bleached and broad shouldered, are mounted on their surfboards at Polzeath beach.

In most other nations there is no doubt to which gender one belongs – there are clear signals of masculine and feminine. Shoes, for instance, are pretty telling in foreign cultures, but just looking at English feet – clad in Dr Martens or heeled, pointed pixie boots – you could be confused as to whom they might belong to. Only here can us British birds be truly adored for our scruffy and unkempt style, or our mouthy masculine sex appeal, while in less enlightened places all that might raise a questioning eyebrow. And only here can we find boys who are comfortable enough in themselves to forgo machismo. Our boys like our girls to be scruffy and tomboyish, and our girls have a taste for boys who are effeminate, expressive and skinny.

No nation takes to androgyny quite like our fair isles. We've been doing it since time immemorial. This isn't really about sexual preference – gay, straight, ambiguous or not, androgynous dressing is about style. For the British bird, sex isn't necessarily top priority when dressing; she uses ambiguity to be cool, not sexy (cool is sexy but sexy is not cool). By dressing androgynously, she is calling out to her mate with very particular signals, different to the usual obvious ones more commonly used when attracting the opposite sex. Her ideal conquest is just as likely to be wearing make-up as she is; she is just as likely to let rip with an obscenity as he is. Oh, happy synergetic English romance.

Some British birds wear skinny jeans and brogues to adopt a masculine demeanour. At the other end of the spectrum, other British birds claim macho points for their unshakeable bravery in the face of English weather. Northern cities on a Friday night in winter will see girls in their bras and bare legs in sub-zero temperatures. Their uncomplicated desire to dress revealingly – despite the freezing chill – becomes macho for the sheer bravado and alcohol it takes to survive the elements in such skimpy attire. That's a different kind of androgyny if you will – boys will be boys but girls will be tougher, hollering at their prey and exuding high levels of testosterone.

Androgynous dressing has also long been a favourite of the upper class, as it allows them to revel in their disregard for the Establishment and middle-class attitudes towards correct and incorrect social behaviour that they often despise. There's nothing like a rollicking good game of crossing the social taboo, display-ing a refusal to choose and a refusal to get bogged down in such mundanities as what gender you might be, loving the confusion and irreverence and the fact that being androgynous somehow makes one truly artistic. Men dressing up in women's clothing at the occasional party tends to be out in the open among the upper and working classes, or more often behind closed doors in the middle classes.

Many an English girl/boy, at some stage in their life, likes nothing more than to be a little bit deviant – stylistically or otherwise, whether you are actually doing the deed or just dress-ing like you might. Deviance is seen as glamorous and, even if frowned upon in public, is secretly widely applauded (look at our tradition of pantomime dames). You can permanently hear our English heroines/heroes utter squeals of delight at all things con-trary and a complete disgust at being expected to be boringly correct. Some of our classiest, most refined characters pride themselves on their inherent wrongness.

Merry England is a thoroughly androgynous society, from Virginia Woolf and her sex-changing literary musings through to Skinhead boys arm in arm with mirror-image shaven-headed, pastel-coloured, braced-up boyish girlfriends (the feminine pastel colours were testament to just how hard the Skinheads were), to the romantic theatrics of the Blitz kids with everyone in make-up and billowing romantic white shirts, to our modern-day insurgence of Indie scruffs.

Oscar Wilde's love of pretty boys culminated in the character Dorian Gray – a horrifically narcissistic spirit, who seduced both men and women of varying social position with his superficial gorgeousness, hiding the grotesque reality of ageing and evil in a painting in the attic. Mr Wilde's was a passionate love of beauty, flamboyancy, androgyny and sadistic wit – and wit is of a piece with androgyny as both are inherently playful.

Can there possibly be a cooler, more culturally poignant image than Mr Morrissey in glass bead necklaces, brooches and oversized, Peter Pan-collared ladies' blouses and flowers? His was an original, masculine but romantic take on women's clothing, a touching comment that summed up a moment in time oozing with a melancholic, anarchic vision. Is that the coolest image of British androgyny? Maybe – but there is a rival in my mind: the image of Vita Sackville-West in her jodhpurs, trilbies, man's jackets and pearls, perhaps expressing a dissatisfaction with the sexual inequality of the early twentieth century, a view commonly shared with her Bloomsbury friends and way before women were accepted into the trouser-wearing community. Vita was the patron saint of Bloomsbury androgyny and perfectly canonised by her girlfriend, Virginia Woolf, who based her hero/heroine Orlando upon her.

But the master of British androgyny is really David Bowie, or Ziggy Stardust, or the Thin White Duke or Aladdin Sane – call him what you will according to your favourite period, he nailed it in all of them. Devilishly handsome, he was the boy who first made English girls fancy men in make-up. Bowie can make anything cool and sexy and credible and sophisticated and render it with an intellectual depth. No matter how weird and wonderful, you can trust Bowie – not even age can harm his seductive powers. Bowie is the ultimate creator of British characters and he goes deep into the psyche of each of his personas. One simply marvels at the Thin White Duke singing 'Stay' and partaking in what looks like a Charleston dance for one of his live performances. It's the coolest, most effortless thing one could ever witness, but his lengthened, heightened poses were obviously constructed with time and obsession in front of the mirror, resulting in a perfect masquerade.

Androgyny does, of course, exist in other cultures, but nowhere so naturally as in England. America, for instance, produces the kind of obvious, fiercely masculine androgyne like Marilyn Manson, all heavy make-up and stripper girlfriend. What is the difference between English and American androgyny? For the Velvet Underground androgyny was something to do with sleaze, but the Rolling Stones used it as a statement: Mick Jagger was beautifully masculine but to that he added an irreverently girlish attitude. No doubt British art schools have a lot to do with this flamboyance and peacockery.

The roll-call of androgynous Brits is a distinguished one: Marc Bolan did it with a top hat, Adam Ant did it with hair accessories and lots of gold buttons, Justine Frischmann did it with a fringe, Vita did it with men's jackets and pearls, Bowie did it with anything from glitter jumpsuits and make-up to a sophisticated wide-leg pant-suit and a trilby. Marianne Faithfull did it with a tie, Sarah Lucas did it with feminism, wit and a grey T-shirt. Pauline Black did it in two-tone suits. Grayson Perry does it in a dress and a raggedly ringletted, traditionally ironic way and makes beautiful and challenging pottery.

Samantha Cameron and Colin Firth are, in their way, thoroughly straight-up-and-down English types. But they are the facade for the riotous (and often darker) deviance that occurs in England. We crave extremes, rebellion, crackpots, prophets, weirdos, outsiders and inconvenient passions far beyond the tidy bounds of straightforward sexuality. We yearn for the kind of wrongness that shatters the mould and doesn't care. That is the real England, the one I try to capture and promote in my work. The fact that it is only seen in glimpses, mischievously hiding behind all that niceness, conformity, respectability and comfortable shoes, makes it all the darker, weirder and more compelling. This is the English genius that I LOVE. It's in the contrast – the working class and upper class, with their talent for the extreme, played off against the neuroses and eerie politeness of the middle class. Tartan kilts and bondage trousers. Prom dresses and Dr Martens.

THE BORROWERS — The effortless English attitude towards androgyny is very practical: it means our versatile Miss Englands get a thrifty kind of two-for-the-price-of-one deal by delving into Mr England's wardrobe. Interchangeable T-shirts and jackets mean you can double your wardrobe strength simply by finding a boyfriend with similar dimensions to yourself. Said boyfriend can be as young or old as you want his clothes to be – if you're looking for jeans a younger more urbane character might be more suitable, tweeds are better from the more mature willowy country gentleman – the Farmer Bean type – or a professor at Oxford. This kind of scheming behaviour might go against one's morals – choosing your partner for his wardrobe pickings in preference to his inner qualities can tug faintly on one's ethics. But one can also pilfer from kin – dad's fishermen's sweaters, coats and tux jackets, grandad's cardies and little brother's blazers are all fair game when it comes to the ancient art of wardrobe filching. The clothes invariably look better, though, if you are actually in love with the provider (especially threadbare sweatshirts), and boyfriends are infinitely the more preferable source of clothes for the simple fact that it is easier to get hold of the said merchandise than from, say, a brother.

Miss England's love of menswear may have been instigated by a French lady (none other than the formidable Coco Chanel) but the clothes she borrowed from her boyfriend the Duke of Westminster were decidedly English – fishing tweeds, Oxford bags and sailing sweaters. She became the master of chic androgyny, powering her sexual allure with male clothes, a petite frame and an acreage of pearls. Back then we had Vita Sackville-West, Virginia Woolf, Dora Carrington and Vanessa Bell – the Bloomsbury women who were all partial to oversized sweaters and jackets worn with skirts and flower prints, giving them a look both rural and intellectual.

These days the difference between English boyfriend dressing and French – for the French seem to glean as much pleasure as us from this pastime – is that the French will always go for a tux, or expensive ripped jeans, and wear it with a load of diamonds and style their hair in a classy up-do and have perfect make-up and look chic and glamorous. Miss E will take her boyfriend's sweatshirt and his jeans, belted and rolled up, and accessorise this with lank hair in a lackadaisical ponytail and no make-up – and look amazing. Miss E might consent to a heel, just as a nod to something more feminine, but the contrary message is clear. In England there is nothing sexier than a beautiful, unkempt girl in an oversized blazer or a dirty parka and an old pair of jeans. It's the way a sloppy sweatshirt hangs off the collar bone, or the way a frayed Turnbull and Asser collar looks slightly too large for a long, feminine neck, or the bunched-up waist of a pair of baggy Oxford bags, or Eighties 501s worn with a white vest, that reaches and attains the sexiest kind of English subversion.

The men's dinner jacket is, arguably, the finest of borrowed attire. Images of toffs spilling out of balls, the girls with squiffed ball dresses, barefoot and covered by a man's dinner jacket, must have inspired the likes of Melanie Ward to wear her own version, forgoing the dress underneath and the accompanying toff. Toffs didn't make good accessories for early Nineties minimalist Grunge. The Eighties were littered with women wearing oversized men's jackets but the best Eighties boyfriend's wardrobe-filchers must be Siobhan Fahey and her Bananarama band-mates. Oversized blazers with the all-important rolled-up sleeves, lumberjack shirts, faded 501s or bus conductor trousers bunched in at the waist with a good thick leather belt. Runner-up prize to Siouxsie, who always made the most of an unstructured black men's jacket, a tie and a waistcoat, adding fishnet and shredded lace into the mix for some fetishistic darkness. Katharine Hamnett, known for her brand of sex and utilitarianism, all with a few Eighties political statements thrown in for good measure, wore her 501 jeans, Chelsea boots and men's jacket or oversized MA1 and made a strong argument for rifling through your boyfriend's sweatshirt drawer. Britpop had Donna Matthews (Elastica) with her fragile, gamine, pixie-like figure in an Adidas tracksuit top and scuffed jeans.

Now we have Phoebe Philo, creative director of the French luxury goods house, Celine, who has developed an incredibly clever eye for the luxury tomboy look – part bourgeois Parisian lady, part English minimalist Grunge boy. Phoebe produces very expensive and beautiful basics, giving a large pinch of extreme luxury to the boyfriend's-sweatshirt-and-jeans look (the jeans are pretty similar to the 501s donned by Bananarama but with meticulous luxury detailing and a hefty price tag). It's a very clever English girl who can sell British tomboy style to rich elite French women.

And one mustn't forget Stella McCartney, who, since she started, has been promoting a pushed-up-rolled-up sleeved jacket with a slim trouser as a succinct testimony to the quintessential Stella-girl, never wavering from the silhouette this gives, and, through such devotion, seemingly perfecting the art of feminine menswear.

We Miss Englands all have an inbuilt tomboyish tendency; we wear high heels but they are more scuffed than a pair of football boots. Girliness also features in the DNA of the British bird, but we like to offset it with a sicker, more mocking element. The more girly we dress, the stronger statement it makes for how silly girlishness is – oversized hair bows and extreme pink make it all a statement of Punk. We Miss Englands are practical by nature and, even if our more experimental side likes to dress up, we must also be able to run, jump, climb trees and get drunk in our clothes – or our interpretations of femininity must look like we have just climbed a tree, complete with bruises and scabby knees.

At the very beginning of my designing career I made a decree that all my dresses must have pockets. Pockets equal nonchalance. I can wear a dress as long as I can stuff my hands in my pockets, thereby affecting the stance of a sullen boy wedging his hands in his jeans. Without pockets one has to stand up straight or hold a clutch bag. I always wanted even the most embellished kind of pumped-up femininity to also express the attitude of a tomboy. Pockets: they seemed the obvious choice.

In all the post-war subcultures, Miss E has embezzled pieces from her boyfriend's wardrobe to mould-breaking and androgynous effect. The Teddy Boy's drape coat looked great with a full skirt and white socks; Mod girls appropriated their beaux's parkas and schoolboy shirts, and Skinhead girls stole their boyfriends' Fred Perrys and copied their boots. Punk groupies ripped off their other 'alves studded leather jackets and seditionary T-shirts – Vivienne Westwood looked her absolute best in a shredded gay cowboy T-shirt and leather jacket and peroxide crop. New Romantics artfully pilfered their gay best mate's Regency shirt and belted it round the waist (Annabella Lwin executed this look perfectly). Sloanes in cocktail dresses wrestled the blazers from their hubbies to warm their exposed shoulders after a rollickingly good hunt ball. Femininity never looks better than when all dressed up in men's clothes, but to accentuate the traditionally feminine has never been our motivation. How could a nation that was brought up on Enid Blyton's Famous Five not want to be the headstrong and terribly courageous character Georgina Kirrin (George) rather than the more delicate Anne (who likes cooking and hates adventures)? The British bird is nothing if not headstrong and up for a good adventure, ginger beer or no.

WHAT DO BRITISH BIRDS LIKE ABOUT ENGLISH MEN?

1) SELF-DEPRECATION — The average British male considers himself lucky if he's able to bag a woman at all. He conforms to that wonderful English cliché and sees himself as the underdog. 'Unlucky,' they shout on the football pitch as yet again he fails to score a goal. The anti-hero; hopeless, hapless, prone to embarrassment, has a stutter, is inhibited and reserved, he is the quintessential English hero.

2) HUMOUR — Above all, the English male will do everything he can to make Miss England laugh. We love him for that.

3) HE'S A SHAMBOLIC DRESSER — The chaotic appearance – mismatched clothes, corduroy or denim depending on age and class – is a style statement in itself. The Army Surplus boots with a Jermyn Street shirt, old cord jacket, girlfriend haircut and stubble – that can only mean he's English. Oh yes, and his winkle-pickers/brogues/brothel creepers, and nondescript trainers. Ultimately, it's his naturalness that breaks hearts.

4) ENGLISH MEN ARE MORE EFFETE — than those of other cultures. From Byron and Shelley to Jarvis Cocker by way of Morrissey, the English affection for the dandy, the fop and the long-haired, snake-hipped male lives on.

5) ENGLISH BOYS LOVE THEIR MUMS — just not in the same way as Italian boys.

6) HIS INABILITY TO HOLD HIS DRINK — three pints and he's anyone's.

7) HE KNOWS HOW — to ride a horse, talk to a dog, operate a piece of large machinery (such as a chainsaw or a tractor).

WHAT DO MEN LIKE ABOUT BRITISH BIRDS?

1) A whiff of the untamed (unhinged).
2) Doesn't mind a bit of mud.
3) She would rather go barefoot.
4) She is quick-witted, frank and disarmingly rude, and gives as good as she gets.
5) She ties her hair up with old rubber bands.
6) She likes jokes.
7) She likes a drink.
8) She has a wicked laugh.
9) She can cook three recipes – brilliantly.
10) She dresses like a boy.
11) She is clever.

GOOD SIGNS IN A MAN — Beard, bad teeth, foppish hair, breeding, odd socks, nail varnish, old Land Rover, guitar, nice suit, boyishness, hair which looks like he's cut it himself, knowledgeable on pop trivia, knows his country code, can light a fire/chop down a tree/put up a tent, good at dad stuff.

BAD SIGNS IN A MAN — Beauty products on his bathroom shelf, talks about his guru/therapist/yoga instructor, has a 'hairdo', wears tight skinny jeans/leather trousers/ironed jeans/anything overtly metrosexual, wears anything by Dolce and Gabbana, pullover slung around the shoulders, coloured Ray-Ban Wayfarers, doesn't know one end of a drill bit from the other.

A SELECTION OF
TYPICAL BRITISH COUPLES

George Harrison and Pattie Boyd

Mick Jagger and Marianne Faithfull

Barbara Windsor and Sid James

Terence Stamp and Jean Shrimpton

Prince Charles and Camilla Parker Bowles

Vita Sackville-West and Virginia Woolf

Justine Frischmann and Brett Anderson

Bobby Gillespie and Katy England

Princess Anne and Mark Phillips

Dylan Thomas and Caitlin Macnamara

Ossie Clark and Celia Birtwell

David Bowie and Iman

Denis and Margaret Thatcher

Vivienne Westwood and Malcolm McLaren

A SELECTION OF
GREAT BRITISH MEN

David Bowie

Brett Anderson

David Hockney

Samuel Beckett

Lucian Freud

Alan Bates

Otis Ferry

Jarvis Cocker

Prince Harry

Ian McCulloch

Morrissey

Joe Orton

All of The Clash
(except, perhaps, for Topper)

Dylan Thomas

Dizzee Rascal

David Sims

John Lennon

Marc Bolan

Withnail

Keith Richards

Malcolm McDowell

TRIBES OF
BRITANNIA

———

So, we know that Miss England's idiosyncratic, erratic style of behaviour starts in pre-school and follows her to the grave. (I want a gravestone covered in shells like the one I saw on a camping holiday in the Outer Hebrides.) So too does her tribal affiliation, or how she defines her sex and status, which comes to fruition in her teens. Part of growing up in England involves the mystical experience that comes with finding one's creative soulmates. One of our most defining national character traits is that we will always cluster into small groups – it's why so many of us desire the bonding that comes with being in a band and why music and bands inspire most of our style. We spend our adolescence rummaging through the vast array of tribes – past and present – that make British culture so fertile and confusing. Even if she is deeply confused – remember, though, confusion is good; it makes Miss E think on a really profound level about her style. Miss E likes mixing old-fashioned status symbols with her own personally contrived, modern – usually meaning retro – ideas of style. Some days she's a Post-Punk Sloane in a pie-crust blouse, blazer and Dr Martens; other days she's an off-duty groupie with unkempt hair and a healthy dose of grungy leopard print, or she will indulge in a nostalgic moment of early Nineties with Birkenstocks and socks. Sometimes it all gets a little too experimental and she looks like she's been dressed by Ziggy Stardust in the dark. However, this could be a good thing depending on the probability of the equation at the time.

The English are a tribe. Stuck on a tiny island (which is probably why we feel more comfortable in small groups), inevitably fighting against the elements and the politics, we are home to rock and roll excess, art-school experimentation and working-class mockery and aspiration. We consistently deliver street style – those youthful aesthetic pretensions – like no other nation. There are two things that one does not talk about in England: class being one, and sex being the other. This is precisely what makes English style so interesting. What we can't express in words we express vehemently in the clothes we wear. The boxes our heritage likes to keep us in can be demolished through intricate clothing combinations that are invented on the street. Style can discuss very complicated cultural issues very clearly and usually blissfully subconsciously. Some girls wear white court shoes because they are ironic (see Alan Clarke's classic Eighties film, *Rita, Sue and Bob Too*); other girls wear them because they think that they're classy. Class is a very important aspect of tribal affiliation. Style can mess with the natural order or it can make those in a particular class, especially the working class, feel like they can fight back against a system that is constantly against them – together as a force, in bondage wear, perfectly cut Crombie coats, bleached denim, gold hoop earrings (the bigger the better). A carefully constructed image never looks better or more like a political attack than when it's multiplied by a thousand and milling around the high street looking intimidating. Subcultures work their best magic when they have a big political or sexual battle to fight.

Similarly, the upper echelons of the class system can show just how posh they reahhly are by going in completely the other direction, looking the most filthy and obtaining the most unwanted items of clothing from the far reaches of Golborne Road. Those in the middle make it much more complicated, either using their chosen tribe to climb the ladder or descend the snake to their desired affiliations, or setting up an array of convoluted style theories based mainly on inverted or just plain normal snobbery. (Many of these people end up as designers or magazine editors.) It must be said at this point that historically the working class is much the best at the tribal thing (the upper class is already defined by how many decrepit castles it owns and the middle class struggles with questioning where it belongs too much). The working class also has much more to fight against and therefore much more to say and fewer ways to say it. The English have realised that clothes are a really good way of expressing yourself when you don't have a lot of money. Your drainpipes can be your castle. Miss E can happily spend most of her weekly wage, without a second thought for food or shelter, on an outfit for Saturday night and use the whole day on a diligent but exultant quest searching for the perfect affirmation of her chosen character for the week.

This is Miss E's dilemma. When everyone around her is a fashion hero/heroine, whom should she follow? Once she has outgrown the natural eccentricities of toddler nirvana, tribal affiliations become serious. Tribes set the co-ordinates of their time; they represent the angst, youthful glamour and social changes of each generation. Even if, more recently, their intricately webbed ideals have been reduced to a bunch of stereotypes, it's impossible to ignore their power. Somewhere between nicking her first obligatory black eyeliner and nail varnish from Woolies (R.I.P.) and getting an honorary membership to the sadly no more Colony Rooms (London's most debauched, cool and elitist drinking club famed for its associations with Francis Bacon and Damien Hirst), Miss E's life becomes a 'style'. She finds a way of resolving the conflict between conformity versus deviance by constructing a way of dressing that has hidden meanings (pink = Punk) and a sense of personal history (ironic *Tatler* girl cocktail dresses = Eighties = HER decade).

These days, pop culture moves at such an astonishing rate that a complex myriad of new subcultures (with their attendant slang/looks/rules) will have been invented – and died – before you've finished reading this ... oops there goes 'Grindie'. Style and tribe are meant to be temporary – a fleetingly brilliant moment in time, guaranteeing its cult status before the new kid takes over. Their ingenuity is mind-boggling. My personal favourite of the moment is the Ganguro. These Japanese girls bleach their hair blonde and wear orange fake tan in homage to our own home-grown Essex girls. Brilliant. Are those clever Japanese things competing for our mantle of irony and eccentric brilliance while we are stuck in limbo with the high street as our own form of style paralysis (sorry, that's a rant for another chapter – see English Classes).

English style democracy concludes that anyone with dictatorial tendencies and an eye for a cheap iconic statement piece can start a sub-tribe and a fanzine (something else the Japanese like about us). In fact, many of these sub-tribes boast less than three members; this is the nature of English elitism – and a very detailed class system of its own. New rules must be invented in order to keep the tribe relevant. No other nation practises the art of belonging (Are you one of us?) so effectively or viciously.

A new consciousness emerges with each new generation that, sweetly, imagines they are the new sliced bread. Where they meet is in the desire to rebel. Where they differ is what they're rebelling against.

The challenge is to create a new look. Who wants to blend in, unrecognisable as the girl in mother's idea of a teenage outfit, when there's a brave new world inspired by Vivienne Westwood? This adventure playground of sedition and perversion has spawned the ultimate English tribe, Punk, which gathers at World's End (Westwood's boutique) at the bottom of the King's Road. Punks are the stuff of fairy tales (Brothers Grimm with Bromley accents). The revered Ms Westwood is, the only designer, apart from Mary Quant and Alexander McQueen perhaps, whose rebellions have stood the test of time and left a definable cultural and political legacy. She offers one of the most important revision tools for Miss E's education and must be studied. Here is a woman who really understands what a tribe is all about, because, put simply, she is the ultimate English 'Mary, Mary quite contrary'.

It's not really about designers, though. Music has had, in my mind, an even bigger part to play in England's obsession with tribalism, from trad jazz through to Echo & the Bunnymen by way of X-ray Spex.

But before Miss E can get her wonky teeth stuck into a tribe, it all comes grinding to a halt. Tribalism, you see, is for the very young (unless you make a career out of it, in which case style-policing authorises access to Hoxton as a 'mature observer'). For Miss E it all starts to make less and less sense, which calls for secretive subversion and real eccentricity. It is time to dismantle and reform tribal affiliations, drawing from nostalgia, personal rebellion and what works on her body. What follows is an interesting period of transition: the twilight of her teenage tribalism and the dawn of her twenty-something brand loyalty. (Are *brand* devotees a tribe?) Swept up in the heady rush of subsequent consumer culture, Miss E struggles to hang on to her spirit of invention; it requires daring and determination. To be frank, for a while there, she might have been lost to the insanity of designer purchases. But she never loses sight of the importance of not becoming a clone, a victim of predictable fashion. She tries to ensure that everything she wears is interesting, which isn't easy when street fashion is absorbed into the mainstream.

Is she no longer capable of stylistic innovation and challenging fashion mores? She wonders if her tribe will survive the ageing process and seem relevant. The insecurity is back. But fear not, Miss E – you are still a BRITISH BIRD.

THE PONY CLUB — If Miss England is a country girl or has middle-class parents with a bit of ready cash, the pony club gives our heroine her first taste of belonging. It's where she learns horsemanship, competition and equestrian fashion: hard hats, jodhpurs, leather boots, hairnets, red and black (Warwickshire) ties, tweed jackets and pale blue Aertex shirts. At pony camp everyone wins; by the end of the day she has twenty red rosettes pinned to her hat. Mucking out horses has a sort of mystic undercurrent. When she grows up she wants to be Jill, her riding instructor with a twenty-a-day Rothman's habit, whose mammoth thighs enfold her mare. Miss E reads books about ponies (graduating from *Black Beauty* to *National Velvet*) and wears her hair in a ponytail. When she attends her first under-11 gymkhana (dressage, show jumping and cross-country), she vows to marry Pudding, her snorting quadruped.

PUNK — This arch, passionate misfit tribe with Carlsberg beer-towels (since banned by the EU) flapping from seats of their bondage trousers, fluffed up in pink mohair jumpers like abused Easter chicks, tore up the rule book and jettisoned conventional ideas of sex. Angry and disillusioned, they deliberately set out to be anti-social. The basic premise of Punk was beautifully, dysfunctionally simple: 'I'm going to make myself so ugly that you will have to notice me.' Punk is the prime example of political struggle leading to great and lasting style; something that modern tribes seem to be lacking.

The Punks stole from the Teddy Boys, borrowing their crepe-soled brothel creepers (originally used for creeping around brothels, obviously) and Brylcreemed DAs (duck's arses), and toughened them up with the leather-trouser-tight-T-shirt combo popularised

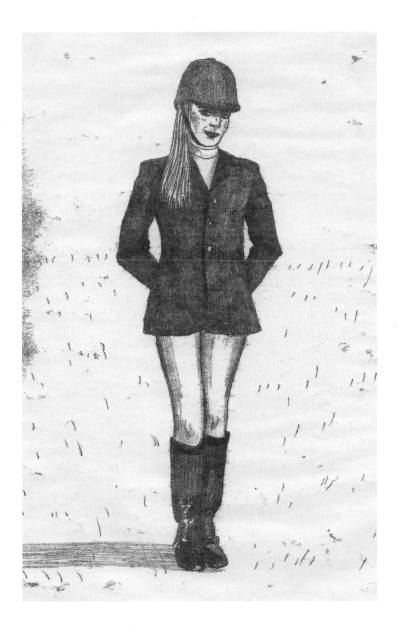

PLATE NO. 26 • THE PONY CLUB

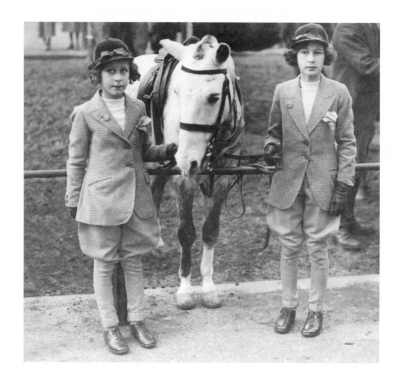

by American rock and roll bands The New York Dolls and The Stooges. Their assault on convention, the combination of anti-authoritarianism and anti-fashion, hit the streets as the rest of the country was hanging out bunting in preparation for the Queen's Silver Jubilee. Punk appropriated the rockers' leather jackets and drainpipes and customised them. It cut up and printed shirts and accessorised with safety pins, bondage straps, studs and bits of string. Cheap, vulgar and utilitarian was good; clothes were made out of PVC, fake leopard skin and bin-liners. Vivienne Westwood and Malcolm McLaren transformed British rebellion with their customised T-shirts, rubber wear and Seditionaries sold from their King's Road boutique, SEX.

PUNK ESSENTIALS

BAND T-SHIRT — The Ramones, Cocteau Twins, Buddy Holly (ironic).

DRAINPIPES — Long before it was possible to buy drainpipe jeans, teenagers borrowed their mums' sewing machines and sewed straight-legged trousers into drainpipes.

BONDAGE TROUSERS — Responsible for the slow shuffle of the Punk, his legs bound in a tangle of straps – and inertia.

MUM PUNK — Chanel rouge-noir nail varnish. Original Blondie T-shirts worn with original Balmain jacket.

GRANNY PUNK — Blue-rinsed old dears under the patron sainthood of British battleaxe Mrs Slocombe in *Are You Being*

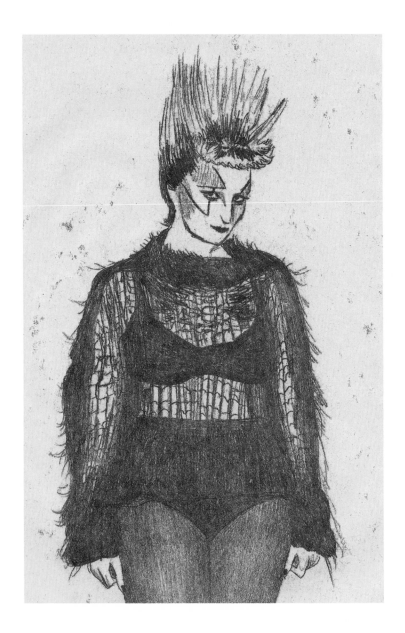

PLATE NO. 28 ∗ PUNK

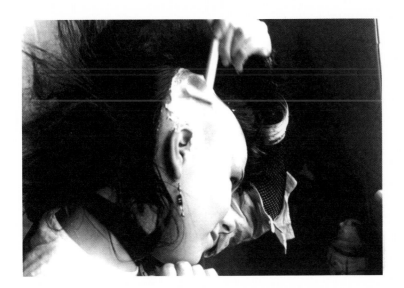

PLATE NO. 29 * PUNK

Served? And arty Hampstead grannies with risqué pink streaks who share a streak of rebellion in the realisation that white hair is dull, and why should old age be boring?

PUNK CHIC — Jet-set glitterati who sport tattoos and partially shaved heads to express an unwillingness to be like mummy (until they land their inheritance) have appropriated the distressed image of Punk; an act of rebellion that is as subversive as modelling for a Mario Testino shoot.

BUFFALO GALS — Buffalo was the prototype of mid-Eighties, West London cool. Even now, there isn't much to match the ideas and unique concepts of Ray Petri and his tribe for their pure, unadulterated coolness – the originality continuously proved by its longevity as the coolest tribe to roam the streets of Eighties London. Petri is the stuff of West London mythology: a stylist who mixed completely disparate, quite bizarre references to create a powerful, sexual, tough street look of French-cut T-shirts, blazers, cheese-cutter caps, cycling shorts, ankle socks and DMs. Did cool even exist before this lot came along? Tribes may have been dissident and full of swagger, but this lot made street style transcendentally heroic as they made their political statement using beautiful mixed-race teenagers, and sublime, but twisted, classicism. The Oxford English could do no better than the simple definition of 'Ray Petri' for its singular definition of the word 'cool'.

Like The Clash before them, the Buffalo group have cemented west London's cultural heritage, even if now it is suffering under the weight of tastefully tasteless rich. For Miss England, congregating outside Finches pub on the Portobello Road will

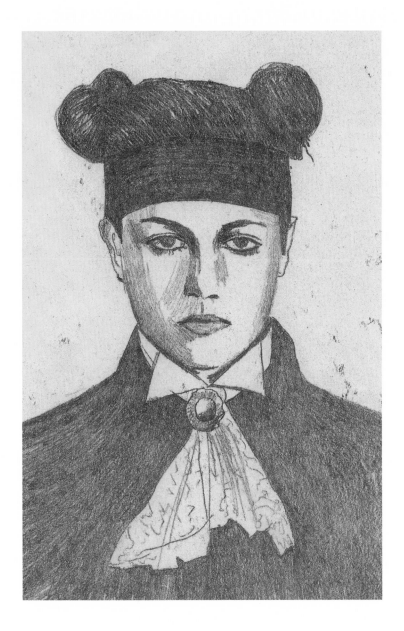

PLATE NO. 30 * BUFFALO GALS

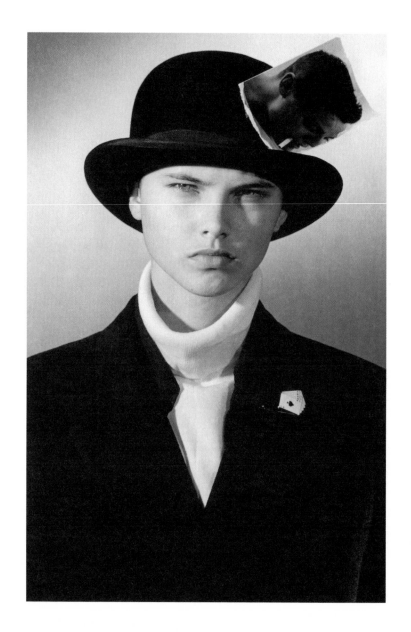

PLATE NO. 31 * BUFFALO GALS

always feel rather like a pilgrimage, and if you squint you can almost see the remnants: lots of black Alaia dresses over leggings, Troop trainers, cheap gold jewellery from Shepherds Bush Market and the ubiquitous MA1 flight jacket, although most of the original group have found Primrose Hill more to their taste in later years. But, if you listen really hard, you can still hear the faint echo of dub and the sweet smell of weed, enough to conjure up an image of Nick Kamen walking down All Saints Road like a W10 Elvis.

GRIME — The chav took label allegiance to such an extreme that all the techniques of subversion that had been passed down from their godfathers like the Mods, Skinheads and Football Casuals seemed lost to bland, zombie-like sincerity and an inane loyalty to one brand. The mockery and therefore superiority to the original had gone. While the chavs seem like sheep, clamouring to the hallowed halls of Burberry like pilgrims to a higher spirit, the emergence of Grime (born in Bow, East London, in 2001) has brought a bit of humour and satire back into the proceedings of working-class style.

Grime has its roots in all sorts of things, taking influences from Jamaica and other parts of the Caribbean, dance hall and hip hop to drum and bass and a little bit of Punk thrown in for good measure. Hoodies and tracksuits admittedly are rife, as are more violent references, but along for the ride are also wit and dandyism, worn on MCs with names like Badness and Bruiser. The Grime kids take casual sportswear ('garms', as these clothes are fondly known) and mix it with designers like Jean-Charles de Castelbajac who is known for his graphic, pop cartoon characters. Grime is very much about the street and urbanity – disaffected

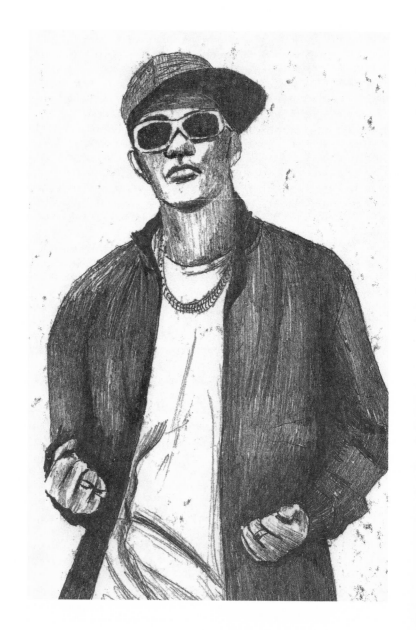

PLATE NO. 32 ∗ GRIME

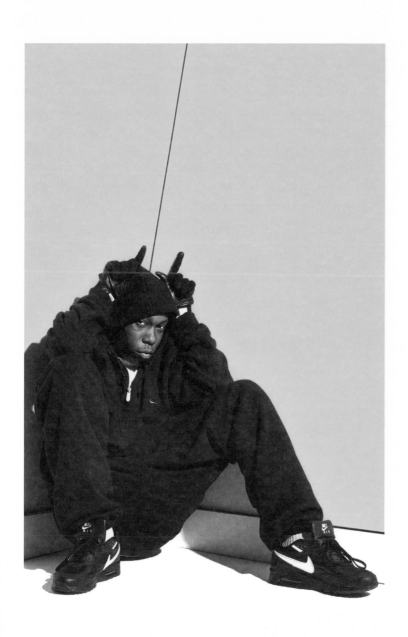

PLATE NO. 33 • GRIME

and alienated British youth on council estates – but it has an inherently British drollness to it and Dizzee Rascal is its mainstream ambassador. One of his successful albums is aptly entitled *Tongue n' Cheek*.

Mr Rascal, like Britain's best street style icons, can take the most bizarre of references – metal guitars and ringtones to Japanese court music – and make it a thoroughly British, random genius affair. Could Grime be the saving grace of sartorial street culture? Only time will tell.

TEDDY BOYS — The originals; the mutinous heroes of post-war British style, the working-class boys and girls who steered Britain on a course of unruly and satirical street style full of bravado and disdain for the Establishment (but also very smart). They were the first to purloin ideas from the upper echelons of the social scale to construct a uniform for a mass working-class youth to aspire and belong to. Clever, intimidating young things.

And, pray, how did they create such a pivotal moment? With an Edwardian suit. Well, a three-quarter-length drape coat and all the trimmings – part Edwardian, part saloon, part Byron – that gave every landlord a kind of laid-back swagger because of the way the length of the jacket made you stand – poised to draw.

This half-velvet-collared jacket first appeared as a flamboyant homosexual look that then evolved to grace the backs of young, upper-class guards officers as a kind of nostalgia for lost grandeur and the era of Edward VII – 'Teddy'. It then carried on its journey down the social scale to the working-class suburbs as high fashion and made for a more intimidating appropriation of the look.

By 1954 it was pure working class with added Western

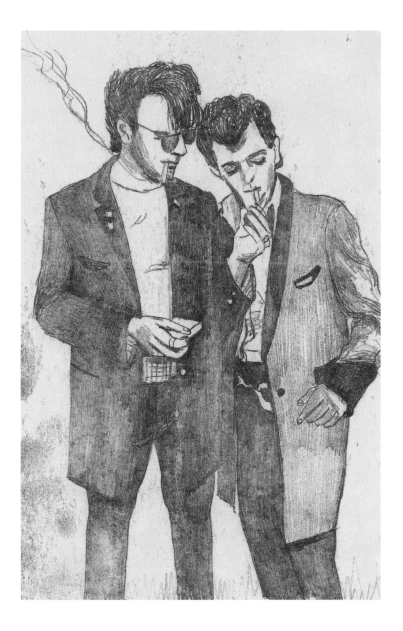

PLATE NO. 34 * TEDDY BOYS

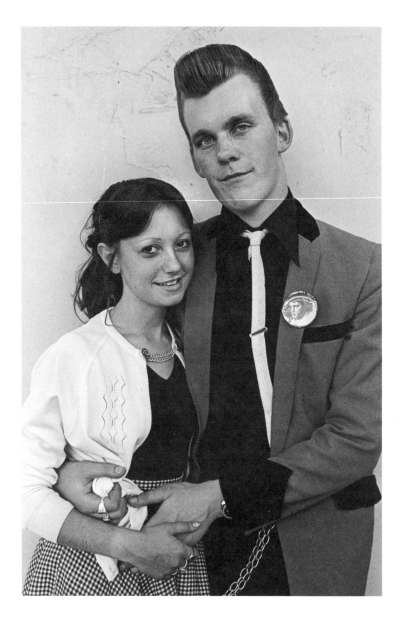

PLATE NO. 35 * TEDDY BOYS

styling – bootstrings with crossbones, eagles and cow-head medallions. Then came the drainpipes, the brothel creepers and the all important hair. The Teddy Boys loved to play with their hair, leaving the National Service short back and sides far, far behind. Crew cuts, spiky tops, the silver dollar, the duck's arse, the square neck and finally the quiff, making the British working class a nation of amateur but very skilful hairdressers.

The first best-dressed Teddy Boy competition was held on Canvey Island, Essex, on August Bank Holiday 1954 and was won by a 20-year-old greengrocer's assistant.

These Teddy Boys and Girls were the first real anarchists – middle-class kids wanted to be them but their parents wouldn't let them. Mass marketing meant that aspirational dressing wasn't a preserve for the wealthy. The working-class kids developed a confident strut and a riotous attitude to their supposed betters – a menacing army of drape-coated boys and leopard-skinned, bobby-soxed, ponytailed girls dancing and fighting to the sounds of rock and roll. By 1957 even Princess Margaret was into rock and roll, tapping her feet elegantly at a Little Richard gig, and so the Teddy Boys, with no other choice, gracefully wound down the most important youth movement Britain had ever witnessed. But there would be more Teddy Boy-inspired anarchy to come.

NEW ROMANTICS — All the anger of Punk and the introspection and polemics of Post-Punk, and a few other finds in the early Eighties supermarket of style and music, could only end up with one susceptible to a moment of culture fatigue. It was time for a bit of gratuitous glamour. David Bowie was again the influence for the New Romantics, along with Roxy Music, and all around one could feel the tension of who looked the most sublime/ridiculous and who could plaster themselves with the most make-up. Music was delivered by Spandau Ballet, The Human League and Visage, all of whom dabbled in excessive amounts of dressing up and costume antics.

This time the music seemed to come second to image. With more electronic-based music and less Indie guitar-led sounds came an increasingly robust club culture, and these club kids paraded themselves around one club created specifically for the movement – Blitz club. These rather brazen characters went on to become the collectively famous Blitz kids.

Boy George and Marilyn were coat-checkers and Steve Strange was the all-powerful decider, leaving a legacy of terrifying door policies that would live on through a whole generation of elitist club doors to come. I missed the Blitz but not the door policy precedent it made: trying to muster up enough self-esteem to get through the doors of the later Kinky Gerlinky was a truly humiliating experience. You had to be tough and severely extreme to tickle Mr Strange's fancy; you had to want it really, really badly – this was elitism and superficiality on a very grand scale.

The New Romantics took a bit of Punk, a bit of English romanticism, a bit of art school (this lot were a St Martins' wet dream), a lot of Glam rock and even more fashion at its most diligent extreme, putting any pretentious catwalk to shame. It was all frills, ruffles, excessive androgyny and heavy make-up, shiny fabrics, big coloured quiffs and swashbuckling costumery. High jinks and high collars after dark. Fun and horror in equal measures.

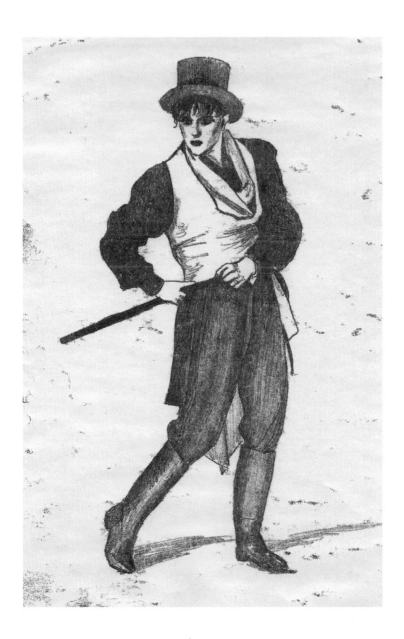

PLATE NO. 36 • NEW ROMANTICS

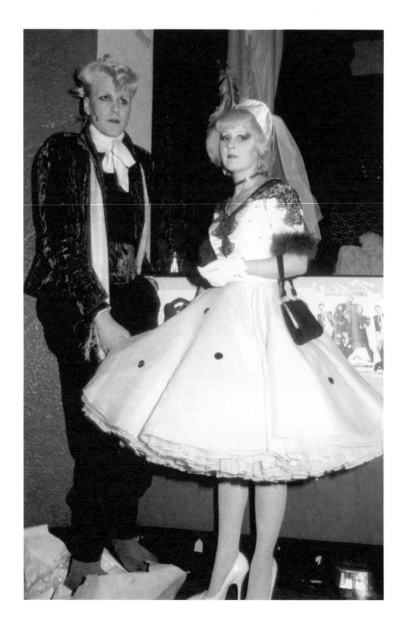

PLATE NO. 37 • NEW ROMANTICS

POST-PUNK — Post-Punk covers quite a lot of ground in my world. First up are the introverted, intellectual experimentalists – the Manchester and Liverpool bands of the late Seventies and early Eighties. The two most influential Ians of our green and pleasant land – Curtis (that dance) and McCulloch (that hair, those lips) – lead the charge into basing music and image on personal feelings. They were both beautiful and highly emotional, as was their music and the way they dressed themselves. Their style was about directing their heads firmly down towards their feet, covered up in greatcoats, trenchcoats and scarves. Joy Division prided themselves on being a band with no image. Nondescript shirts, trousers and second-hand clothes. Heavy, dowdy pieces from army and navy – a kind of refugee look – accessorised with a little satchel or a duffel bag; all looking quite post-war but also with a huge nod to Mr Bowie. A lot of Post-Punk was an extension of the artistic sensibilities of the outré music of the late Sixties and Seventies.

Punk (the wayward father) was about an intimidating look, expressing your anger and trying to rock the Establishment with speedy, uncomplicated, nihilistic music and similarly punchy fashion statements. Post-Punk was more introspective and brooding. As soon as Punk became a recognisable formula, which pretty much took the usual lifespan of any tribe (two years or thereabouts), the people who had been inspired by the first round took the seeds of Punk and mutated them, trying it from other angles. Punk gave way to Post-Punk which, in my book, grew into the most radical, forward-thinking music and fashion ever made.

Post-Punk was intelligent and imaginative, and on the surface less about the clothes (although their collective look was as instantly recognisable and as affected as its predecessor; only

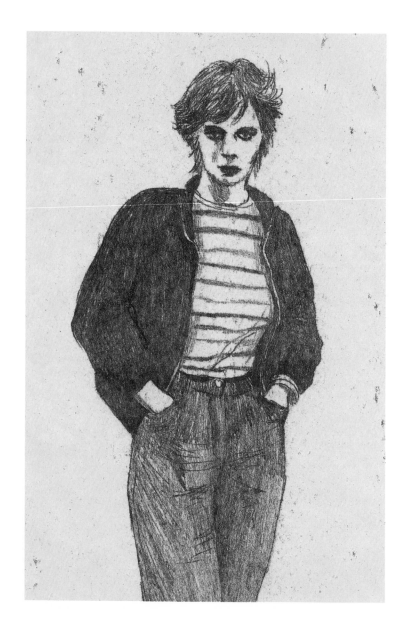

PLATE NO. 38 • POST-PUNK

it screamed of tortured talent and feeling as opposed to hedonistic antagonism). The clothes all looked like old people's clothes – your auntie's cast-offs like raincoats. (Ahh, The Raincoats.)

The likes of Joy Division, Echo & the Bunnymen, Gang of Four and Julian Cope were essentially industrial poets, taking their drab surroundings and their interest in art, politics, literature and, of course, music and turning them into a strong, heartfelt image. They may have shunned fashion but in its own way this was the most brilliant, pretentious minimalist style one could create after Punk. Anti-style never looked so cool and this was a really clever, moody group of people with a Kafka novel firmly shoved under one arm.

There were many more bands that would dance to the ethereal tune of doom and gloom – Orange Juice (Edwyn Collins pursued a charming, accidental and very un-rock-and-roll look of sandals, Oxford bags and make-up that can't have been easy in Glasgow and made for a strong statement that was all rock and roll in the true sense of British rebellion), Josef K, Aztec Camera, The Bluebells – usually deriving from Northern cities and Postcard or Factory records, but none summed up the aching mood quite like the two Ians. You could be forgiven for thinking Punk was all about white working-class boys from London. Post-Punk was about different areas and ultimately a different sex.

And what a group of iconic females they were. From Siouxsie to The Raincoats via Jeanette Lee (PiL) and Clare Grogan (Altered Images). My very favourite kind of girls.

While Punk gave empowerment to women, albeit a kind of eye candy in fishnet tights and stilettos, Post-Punk saw the modern rock and roll woman let loose and there was surely a strong pinch of feminism and androgyny in the mix of the ultimate Post-Punk girl or boy. Never before had the boys' club that was rock and roll been so infiltrated by women as equal participants – producing eclectic, riotous melody and equally eclectic and riotous outfits, both of which played ambivalently with ideas of what hipness and coolness were – just like Edwyn in Glasgow.

Their music questioned a lot of things – the importance of romantic love, gender, racial and economic inequality – and all this was perversely dressed up in vintage dresses and beribboned hair. The message always goes down best with a good melody and an equally good look.

These women were revolutionaries: Ari Up aged 14 wearing her knickers over her bobbly, thinning black tights, and The Slits chanting politicised lyrics in tulle rah-rah skirts and homemade T-shirts; Poly Styrene with bows in her hair, prim vintage cardies, pretty jewellery and tin army hats and chunky braces on her teeth. I particularly love the way she played with the idea of ugliness and used it as her power and charm. Pauline Black and her androgynous tonic suits; Jeanette Lee in romantic Victorian pedalpushers and baggy second-hand jumpers; Clare Grogan in cocktail dresses, Capri pants, ankle socks and ballet slippers and the obligatory fabric tied around her head. The Raincoats sang jagged songs about being no one's little girl in little vintage dresses, necklaces and denim jackets. Or Bananarama, although sadly better known for their Stock Aitken Waterman period of pop, who started life as tomboys doing their first demo with a few of the Sex Pistols, following that with a spot of backing vocals for Iggy Pop and The Monochrome Set.

English style is at its best when it takes its cue from music or larger cultural experience rather than simply what a designer

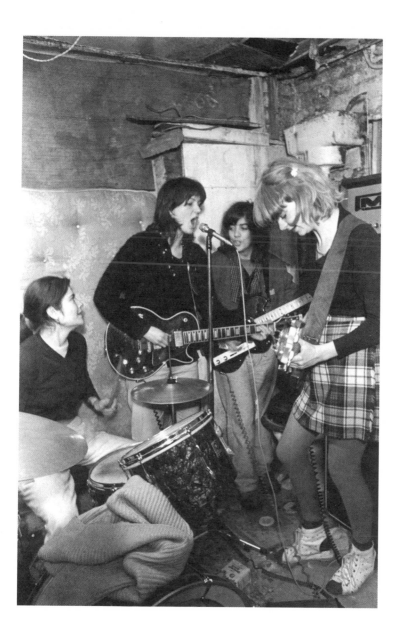

PLATE NO. 39 * POST-PUNK

says, and this is something – although a designer myself – I have always tried to incorporate into what I do in my day job.

Post-Punk, New Wave girls were all groundbreaking devotees of second-hand clothes and eclectic styling, and all these girls have completely inspired the Luella brand, because Luella was never about purist, dictatorial looks. It was always about a celebration of English girls and culture and music and individualism. It mixed styles and ideas and found things and new ideas, taking inspiration from the way the Post-Punk women wore their clothes; never about money, but character. Not even really about fashion but about pieces that clothed and enhanced an attitude and a fantasy and a strange femininity. Avoiding sexuality as a currency or an enforced chicness because the Post-Punk girl, and in turn the Luella girl, was never about that, she was never a ten-foot-tall skinny model, she was more fun: rich in the head, not in the pocket. The Post-Punk girls have always been the ones I have looked to for that all-important English attitude to style.

GRUNGE — The Eighties was a busy time for an experimental and ultimately rather brazen Miss England, no matter what sex or class she happened to be flirting with.

In the Nineties Miss E crashed and burned. And what an exciting time that was. This was that very special moment when Miss Moss came out for all those gawky Miss Es out there who didn't look like Cindy Crawford or Claudia Schiffer. A cute and very cool imp with the best laugh in England wearing greying cotton knickers and a vest in a suitably down-at-heel location.

Kate became an instant icon, her waif looks fitted perfectly with the militant shift, but she also had a personal style and incredible charisma; she was great at putting clothes together which made this new character instantly believable.

Kate was raw, gritty, innocent, sexy, street and militant all at the same time. She wore her hair lank and parted at the centre (thanks, Guido), floor-length denim skirts and socks and Birkenstocks and random flea market bits that Melanie Ward would find and then customise.

David Sims with his shoots in *i-D* and *The Face*, and Melanie Ward and Anna Cockburn making the clothes he would shoot, created a new spirit for Miss E to love and cherish still to this day. Cockburn's silver leggings seem particularly relevant.

David, Melanie and Anna dismissed the very perfect, Amazonian, glossy, maximalist bodies that were prevalent at the time and found gawky teenagers and played with the idea of gangly and ugly, making bow legs and pigeon toes and goofy imperfection something of beauty – an outsider beauty that had a deeply seductive charm winning over a generation. Theirs was a proud rebellion, and they had an ardent admiration of the underdog and the unique imperfections that make people and outfits beautiful. Melanie gave it innocence and romance; David gave it a harder-rock and roll edge; Anna gave it an ironic, intellectual stance.

This was new and different and anti everything. All it took was a few dissatisfied, talented people to completely change the landscape of British style; in fact, turning it on its heels and marching it in the opposite direction.

Okay, so Grunge wasn't an entirely British invention. Some credit must be given to a band from Seattle. Kurt Cobain was as an incredible icon as can be and wore a great plaid shirt, perfect ripped jeans and made me for one appreciate the subtlety of a bad peroxide job. But stylistically that was about it. There was Courtney Love in satin slips, tiaras, tattoos and smudged lipstick

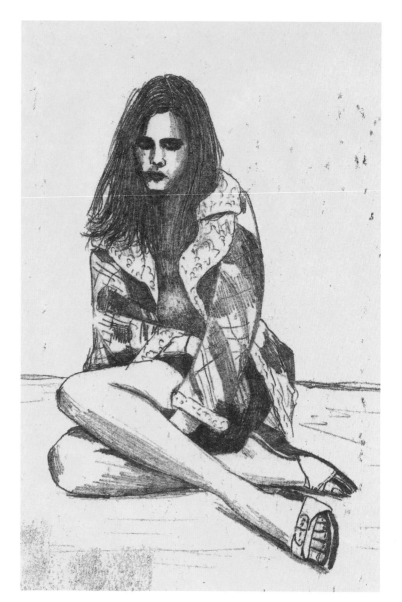

PLATE NO. 40 * GRUNGE

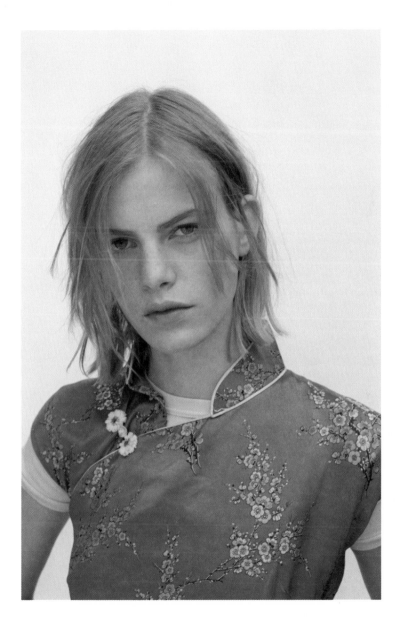

PLATE NO. 41 • GRUNGE

(rather too obvious for a nation of Miss Es with generations of sartorial elegance to look back on). We English embraced the politics and the ideas of Grunge, then tweaked it and refined it and gave it style and a grubby parka.

GLAM(ROCK) — Obsessed as I am by androgyny and cross-dressing, women in men's suits and men with girls' haircuts, I hereby dedicate this section to skinny, glitter boy David Bowie, who seems to have inspired at least half of the tribes in this chapter. Stealing from transvestitism, outer space, old-fashioned Hollywood glamour, the Twenties and mime, Bowie interchanged elements of masculine and feminine dress and produced a sort of flamboyance. Ziggy Stardust was the hero of the Glitter Revolution; he made it okay for everyone to wear mascara. Bowie puts it best:

Everything we knew was wrong. Free at last or, if you like it, at sea without a paddle, we were giving permission to ourselves to reinvent culture the way we wanted it. With great big shoes.

The Seventies would not have been complete without Tim Curry doing the time warp as Dr Frank-N-Furter in 1975's *The Rocky Horror Picture Show*. His muscular rooooooooOOOOOAR in fishnet stockings was a revelation. He was part of the preamble to the Eighties New Romantics, that foppish tribe of androgynous weirdos who favoured frills and make-up *en hommage* to the English Romantics.

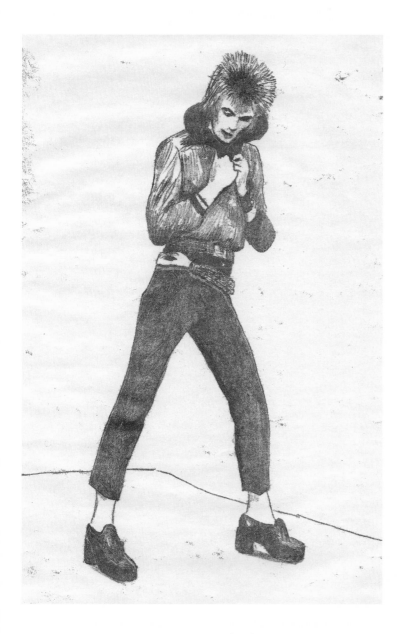

PLATE NO. 42 * GLAM(ROCK)

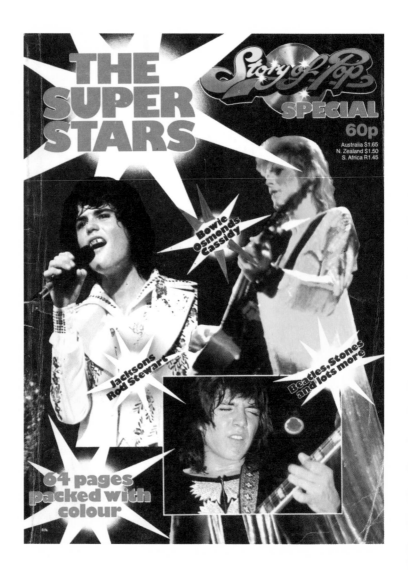

M O D S — Before we had chavs, we had the stylistically superior Mods and Skinheads, their hardcore younger brothers. Sixties Mods were well-turned-out, detail-obsessed, working-class boys and girls whose *raison d'être* was to be fashionable, to be modern and to look sharp in well-cut Italian suits with narrow lapels and tapered trousers, thin ties and winkle-pickers. Suits were purchased from men's tailors such as Burton and John Collier or the new boutiques on Carnaby Street owned by John Stephen. I sat in a cab the other day and when I asked the driver to take me to Arnold Circus (in Shoreditch, where my studio resides) he gave me a guided tour back in time to where he hung out as a Mod and parked his scooter along with hundreds of others round the corner outside Shoreditch town hall. He also told me about how he ordered a suit from a Savile Row tailor that took him two years to pay off. Every Saturday he would go to the shop and give another chunk of his hard-earned wages – his only deposit was the good word of his father.

In their revivalist Seventies incarnation, Mods adopted two-tone shiny suits inspired by Jamaican Rude Boys, Harrington jackets (black or maroon cotton zipped jackets with tartan linings), maroon Sta Prest trousers, Ben Sherman and Fred Perry twin-tip polo shirts, army-green parkas and Crombie overcoats.

S K I N H E A D S — Skinheads emerged from the split in the Mod movement in the Sixties and were initially known as 'hard Mods'. They emerged as the aggressive counter to the Sixties glamorisation of youth and adopted the Ska and reggae from South London's Rude Boys. They adopted a uniform look of cropped hair, red braces, Crombies, turned-up Levi's (white or denim) and polished, 14-hole Dr Martens monkey boots or brogues with white

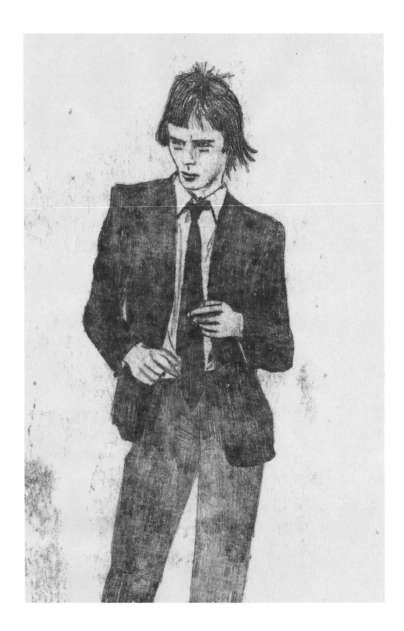

PLATE NO. 44 • MODS

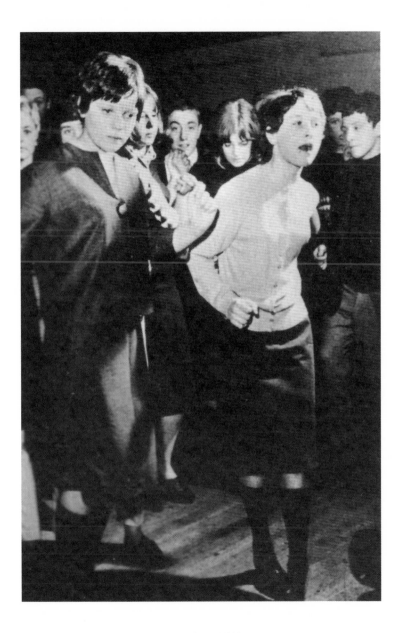

PLATE NO. 45 * MODS

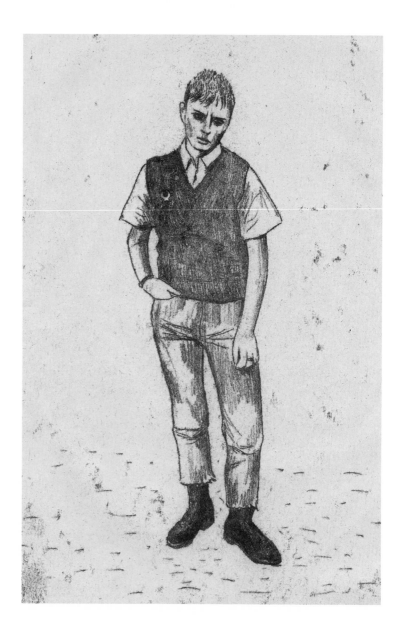

PLATE NO. 46 * SKINHEADS

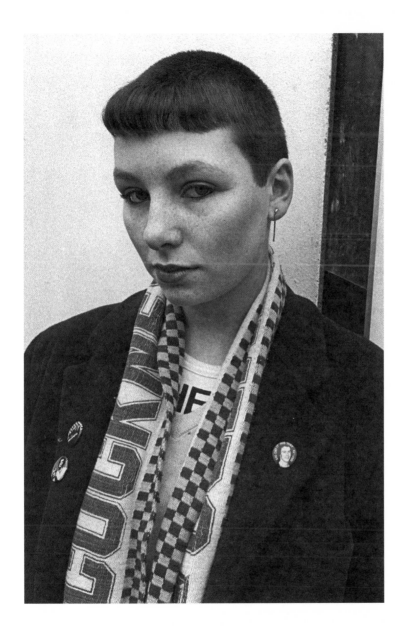

PLATE NO. 47 * SKINHEADS

socks. Skinhead girls wore faded (bleached jeans) with one-inch turn-ups, red braces over checked Ben Sherman shirts and polished Dr Martens. It was said that you couldn't tell them apart unless the girls were wearing miniskirts with fishnet tights. Skinheads were aggressive in their need for self-expression at a time of growing anxieties about class and joblessness; this was the alienated working class retribalising itself.

S K A — Ska originated in Jamaica in the late Fifties with the arrival of the radio, enabling Jamaican artists to hear rhythm and blues and, in turn, record their own versions.

Fast forward to the late Seventies in the rather disheartening confines of Coventry and the birth of the English 2 Tone revival. Bands like The Specials, The Beat, The Selecter (see Pauline Black also in Post-Punk) took the original sound of Ska and added faster tempos and a harder edge to make a kind of heady Reggae/Punk concoction. The socially conscious Specials arguably lead the movement (although the heroes of the legendary Clash before them were influenced by the Reggae they heard in West London) writing songs about the state of the country and the gloomy picture that was an integral part of their adolescence – Thatcher's Britain: riots in Liverpool, recession and unemployment. They sang mini kitchen-sink dramas illustrating just how dismal the times were. Songs about teenage pregnancy ('Too Much Too Young') and depicting the grim sights of once inspiring cities with no life left in them ('Ghost Town') summed up a colourless life for Eighties teenagers. 'Man at C&A' depicted a state of no hope. (Although I clearly remember a time spent shopping in C&A with my mum. Clockhouse was where it was at in 1984 when I was ten years old, but I can see how it might look slightly more apocalyptic to a dissident teenager from Coventry.) Though the inspiration was a harsh reality, it didn't stop Ska being the easiest, most uplifting music to dance to and had skinny-tied teenagers bouncing like they'd never bounced before – not pogoing but a progression to rhythmical bouncing. An elevating kind of 2 Tone.

Ska was seen as a racially unifying youth movement, even though, at times, it attracted a right-wing Skinhead element. The West Midlands had the highest population of black people in England and the youth clubs and discos had a strong Reggae bent. Ska was almost inevitable. Working-class black and white musicians who had grown up together, been at school or worked in factories with each other now formed bands together and constructed a slick, strict uniform of black suits, white shirts, white socks, skinny ties and pork pie hats and trilbies. (2 Tone was a big influence on my early collections.) Terry Hall of The Specials said it was actually the *Guardian* newspaper that pointed out The Specials were a multi-racial band, 'but it just felt natural to us'.

Jerry Dammers was the real genius behind the creative direction of Ska. He produced the image both on and off paper, creating the 2 Tone record label complete with homemade graphics and compiling the Ska look from second-hand shop finds and being particularly stringent in his opinions of the exacting image of the band. Fights would ensue about whether a defiant band member would stand up to Jerry's single-minded vision and wear the white T-shirt instead of the white shirt – typical English street style perfectionism and minor rebellion.

The undiminished pleasure of jumping up and down to Eighties Ska band Madness was confirmed at 2009's Glastonbury. Suggs, ever the gent, was pink-shirted with a matching pink handkerchief adorning his top pocket (a dying art).

PLATE NO. 48 * SKA

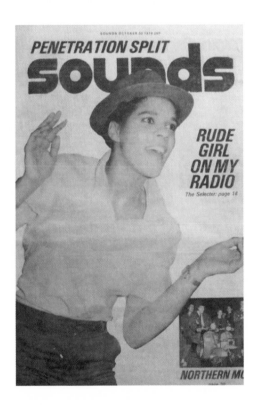

PLATE NO. 49 * SKA

CASUALS (AKA MATCH LADS) — These early Eighties football fans originally hailed from Liverpool and adopted David Bowie's androgynous wedge haircut seen on the cover of the album *Low*. Casuals' floppy girlish fringes, tight Lois jeans and trainers were deemed effeminate and therefore revolutionary for boys. In the label-obsessed Eighties, they evolved a look that revolved around a fondness for expensive sportswear and designer labels. Their brief was to look smart (pukka) in Sergio Tacchini, Ellesse, Fila and Lacoste shirts, jackets and shoes. They adopted a preppy tennis chic that extended to designer labels Armani, Burberry and Aquascutum. Influences were as diverse as *The Two Ronnies* and Björn Borg.

GOTHS — 'Does it come in black?' When you consider that Goths were a nomadic warrior people who inhabited the forests of northern Europe in the third century, you realise how far we've come. You can't open a style publication without seeing what's commonly referred to today as 'Goth,' i.e. black. The gloomy, macabre image of Goth is a stalwart of fashionable winter garb. Goth is modernity's 'other' with its associations of sorcery and witchcraft; it symbolises dark romance and rebellion. The Gothic subculture grew out of Punk, and drew on Gothic literature. Their music was marked by introspective lyrics and synthesisers. Siouxsie Sioux was, and perhaps remains, the queen of elegant Gothic gloom.

Today's Gothic subculture is associated with black-clad teenagers who cluster outside fast food restaurants – black is how they feel. Or is rather less provincial when adopted by French fashion editors and designers who have pushed the look away

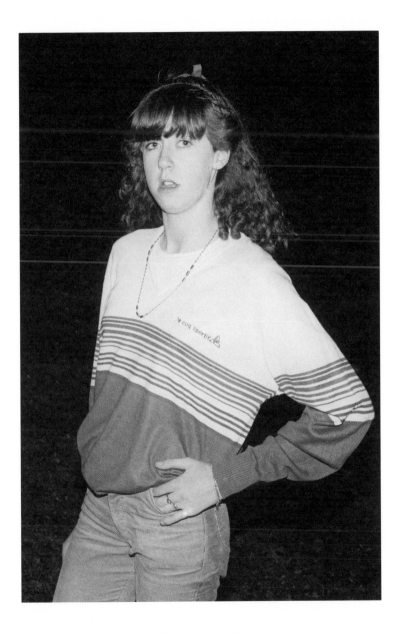

PLATE NO. 50 ∗ CASUALS

PLATE NO. 51 * CASUALS

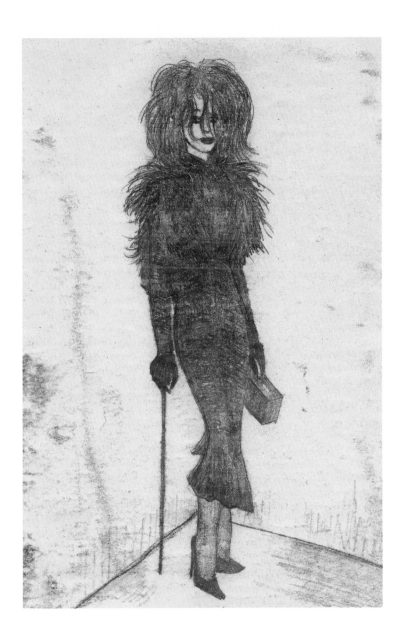

PLATE NO. 52 * GOTHS

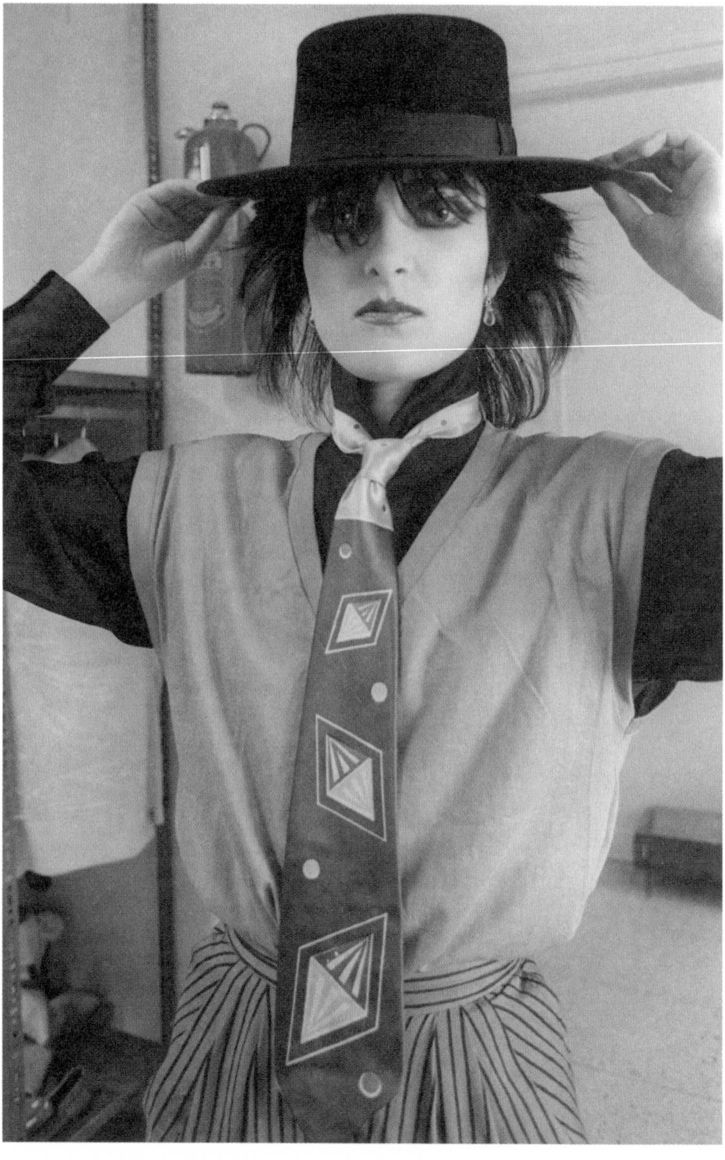

PLATE NO. 53 • GOTHS

from shapeless, elasticated-waist purple skirts and into sharp and sexy black, figure-suffocating territory.

Distinguishing between Gothic sub-tribes is crucial to grasping their essence. Traditional Goths wear Victorian-style long coats and old vintage dresses. Cyber Goths (very into technology) wear latex, rubber, lots of PVC, and dye their hair all sorts of rather bright colours.

Baby Bats are 2010's Gothic Lolitas, a Japanese sub-tribe and one of my favourites for their vintage dresses and girlish morbidity. The Japanese embrace English subcultures with fanatical passion, holding up a mirror to our own eccentricities.

The legacy of Eighties Goths (besides liquid eyeliner) is the ubiquity of black, which is associated with the fashion world, executive women and rebellion. Barbara Hulanicki couldn't find a simple black dress so designed one herself. Mary Quant faced the same dilemma, and acted accordingly. The Queen, on the other hand, can't wear black unless she is in mourning.

E M O S — Emos, like Goths, are very popular in the far reaches of provincial England (especially Cornwall – I like spotting them on the beach reading and looking a bit hot). These emotional, Punky, Indie creatures hide behind long dyed-black fringes, lots of red and black eyeliner, skinny jeans and slightly orthopaedic-looking chunky skate shoes. Into poetry, they think Evanescence is great. The varying severity of the condition 'Emo' is proportionate to how scoffed at they are.

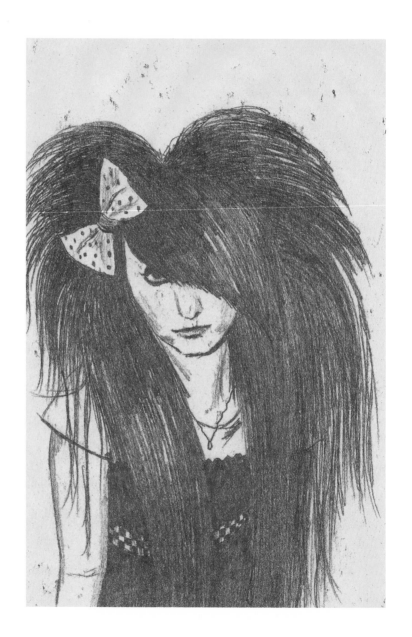

PLATE NO. 54 * EMOS

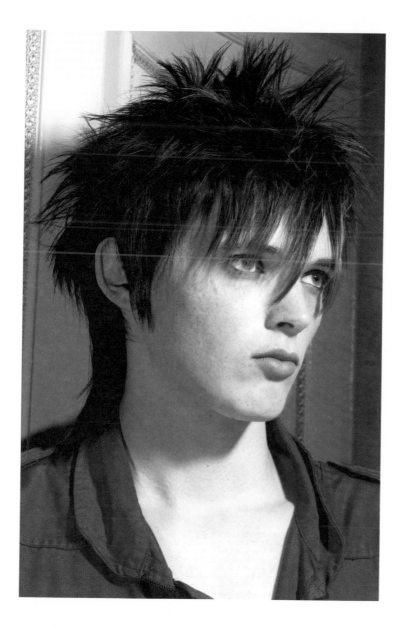

PLATE NO. 55 • EMOS

SLOANES — The fundamental rightness of having a Peter Jones account, wearing dad's Pringle jumpers and putting baked beans into the shepherd's pie remains unchallenged. Art courses at the Courtauld and a couple of years at House of Hanover are followed by a fledgling marriage to Charles.

Princess Diana personified the Eighties Sloane in her high-necked frilly blouses, pearls, loose three-quarter-length skirts, pumps and Rimmel blue eyeliner. A traditional English rose, she was pleasingly curvy with a creamy complexion. This all changed, of course, with the divorce and her bid for freedom so that by the mid-Nineties she had become *the* so-called New Sloane: ultra-groomed, tanned, Versace-clad. Despite being a rebel (attending a Buckingham Palace tea party bare-legged), she never abandoned her uniform of upturned collars, denim and pearls (and sunglasses worn like a tiara).

Sloanes personify the English approach to good manners, which is to ensure the dog is fed before enjoying a cup of tea and *The X-Factor*. This is where Britain's upper and middle classes meet. It extends to a shared taste for Heinz baked beans, instant coffee (Nescafé) and custard creams. Sloanes discuss dogs rather than their children and are good at fun: practical jokes, smutty jokes, fancy dress balls (this is particular to toffs) and silly nicknames. What they hate is anyone trying to be *clever*. They are avowedly anti-intellectual and can't abide anyone taking him/herself too seriously. 'Oh don't be so *boring*,' is a popular Sloane put-down – unless he writes a column for the *Daily Telegraph* or has a seat in the Lords and is therefore allowed intellectual pursuits over heartiness.

The scruffy Sloane (conspicuously frayed collar, coat covered with Labrador hairs, muddy Aigles, scuffed brogues) is acceptable among men. Women must tidy up in town but may be dishevelled at home in the countryside (Gloucestershire).

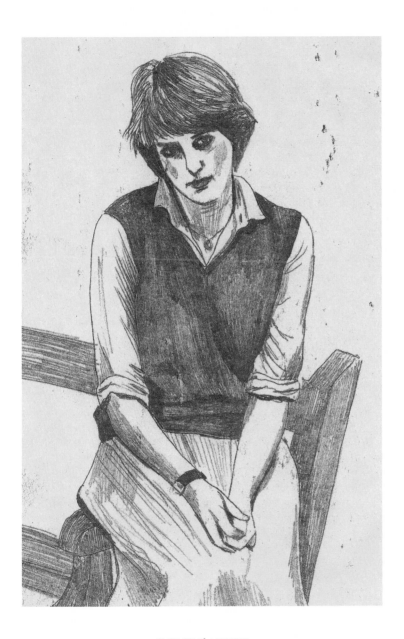

PLATE NO. 56 • SLOANES

My Sloane is the Eighties Sloane. The rigidity of her uniform and the rules by which she lived deserve to be preserved. Sloanes wear red, white and blue to fly the flag, announce their loyalties and stick to what they know. Blue is regimental, nautical and goes with everything. Navy tights mean business. Red is jolly. White is the colour of school shirts and the snow at Verbier.

SLOANE STAPLES

PIE-CRUST BLOUSE — A variation on the ruffle, this is the Sloane's romantic nod to Victoriana. It adds prettiness to the V-necked jumper; an alternative to plain white or a rugby shirt.

BALLET SLIPPER — By French Sole or Bally or Ferragamo, the low-heeled black patent pump is non-threatening, ensuring that the Sloane isn't taller than Charles.

HAIRBANDS — The safety of the velvet hairband can't be underestimated. It means that the Sloane can light a Silk Cut, floor the Merc and make weekend plans on the hands-free phone. It also means that she looks like mummy, and everyone at school, and Aunt Penelope.

BLAZERS — A classic, as easy to slip on as the old school blazer. They combine detail (crests, gilt) with sharp tailoring and a sense of purpose (regatta, cricket, tennis).

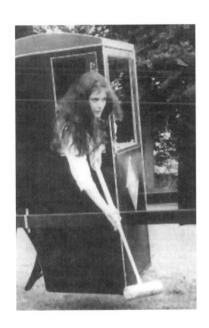

PLATE NO. 57 • SLOANES

WEST LONDON ARISTOS — Being from honourable descent gives a certain confidence and inherent ability to wear crap and still look both stylish and slightly noble – see English Classes chapter. The market stalls around Portobello that hold the filthiest clothing debris have a strange magnetic pull to anyone with a posh, usually second generation bohemian background, for whom dressing in the most unwanted textile rubble on the far reaches of the Golbourne Road is considered the height of sublime refinement. Posh people elsewhere in the capital seem to adhere to a fairly standard rulebook that, although subtle, still sticks to the correct snobbery protocol. In W10 it is quite to the contrary – a very exclusive tribe indeed.

In the same way as those working class kids who wear all their wealth on their chests, this lot, who invariably live in-between Notting Hill and the Harrow Road and have decaying, cluttered family piles/unconventional retreats in Wales or Ireland, wear their inherent dispassion for status symbols on their moth-ridden, irony-laden sleeves. The only way to distinguish one of these tribes from the genuine unfortunates that parade up and down Westbourne Park Road is the occasional piece of inherited couture – an old Balenciaga jacket disguised heavily by the non-descript anorak over the top and tracksuit pants underneath. The West London Aristo is often without ready cash, as most jobs are considered as gratuitous as new clothing unless it's a pastime that involves archiving something for a friend's dad or a job that involves shopping for records on Portobello Road. W1 is only really frequented after dark and usually on a Thursday for Gazza's Rocking Blues in a medley of strange vintage prints and mother's original Sixties lamé, but never for a trip to Selfridges – oh the shame.

Bohemia has had mixed press over the last few years, not helped by the commercialisation of the original West London

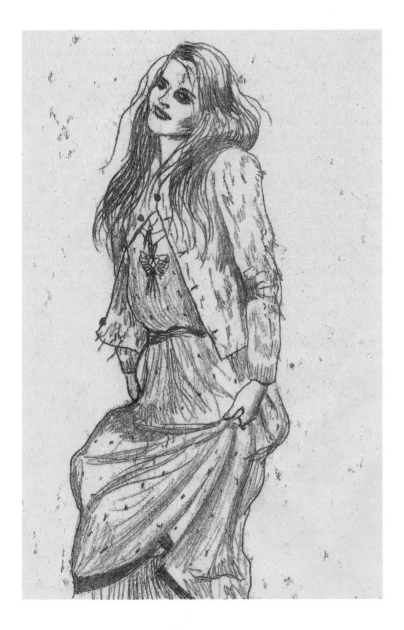

PLATE NO. 58 • WEST LONDON ARISTOS

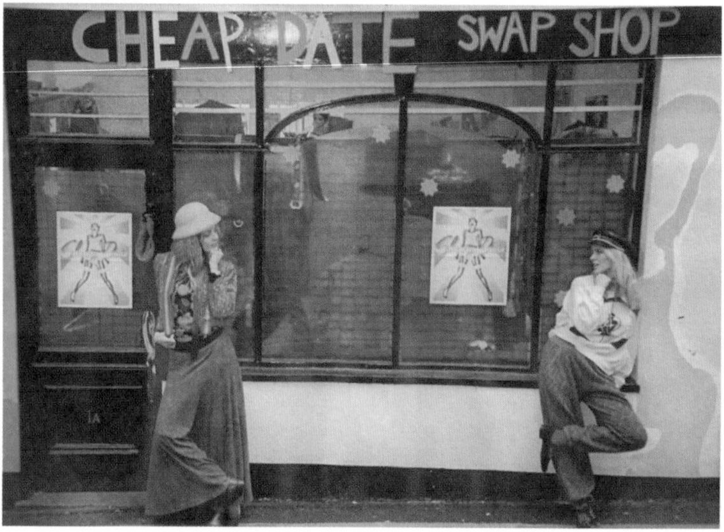

PLATE NO. 59 * WEST LONDON ARISTOS

bohemian who is actually quite smelly, cold, and now – by the more sanitised offshoots – blonde actress types in fringing. But the true aristocratic bohemians that loiter around decaying town houses at the upper end of Portobello are really something to be marvelled at. The genuine article is actually a special kind of creative, unhindered by class insecurity and happy to cast themselves completely adrift from any kind of fashion or beauty code of behaviour. It's all about confidence. Not everyone in this tribe has impeccable, blue-blooded bohemia running through their veins, but there is a general feeling of privileged style deviance and militant contrariness.

The genius behind this tribe comes in the form of a fanzine/manifesto. Its creator, Kira Joliffe, gives what could be a load of posh girls in tea dresses and cashmere a bit of edge, depth and wit with her ode to charity shopping, *Cheap Date*.

But it is the previous generation that really invented the idea of aristo rebellion, culminating in leaving London altogether in a convoy of gypsy caravans to rural fairyland.

Some though – as with most tribes – can fall into stereotype. For those, a cautionary tale …

While Daisy was doing her A levels, Daisy's boyfriend broke in and stole mummy's diamonds. Byron got six months: Daisy got three Ds, which almost stopped granny passing on her entire collection of Dior couture and her flat in Bassett Road, while she decamped to the annex of Uncle Ned's extensive pad in rural Italy. Daisy's going to stay true to her promise of a month's rehab in Arizona, while Byron is held at Her Majesty's pleasure. True story with names changed to protect the guilty.

RAVE — Warehouses in the dark corners of London, the legendary Haçienda in Manchester, secret Sunday afternoon clubs and muddy Sussex fields were the ticket to freedom – and friendship – in a most un-English way. Rather like having to shake hands with your neighbour in church. After the frilly self-consciousness of New Romanticism and the electronic pantomime bands that accessorised it, electronic music progressed into clubs and into the hands of DJs, via the genius behind New Order – Blue Monday was one of those singles that just summed up everything really. The end product, Acid House with its baggy T-shirts, dungarees and long hair, was a breath of fresh air, although actually the air invariably smelled of stale alcohol and cigarettes and sweat and loved-up, drug-addled, facially-morphed people who looked much more terrifying than any aforementioned Goth. All-night dancing meant trainers: Travel Fox, Adidas Stan Smith, Nike Airs. Hot clubs encouraged the wearing of baggy trousers, leggings, Lycra and lots of white to dazzle under the UV. Boy George and Jeremy Healy's E-Zee Possee's 'Everything Starts with an E' was the bittersweet anthem for the latter half of the Eighties with its sinisterly happy football hooligans, girls in their underwear and boys in smiley face T-shirts. Looking back on a tribe that I have first-hand experience of, I realise, when considering style anyway, it really was rather awful. More interesting, stylistically and musically, were the Rave/Indie kids who came out of Manchester and Factory records a few years post-New Order – The Stone Roses, Happy Mondays. For all the sunken-cheeked grey complexions, it felt like something morosely poetic and romantic – the contrariness of these rather rough-looking boys with moronic dance steps creating brilliant music.

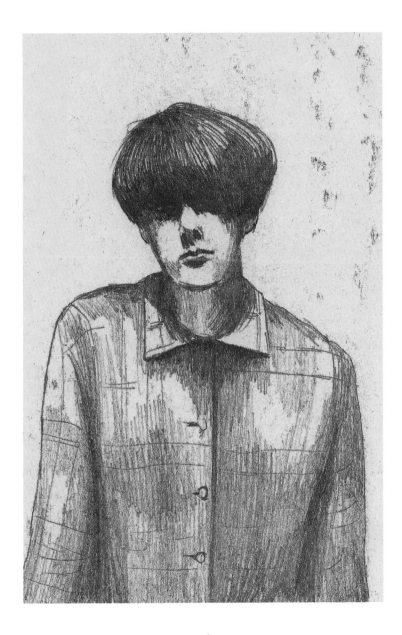

PLATE NO. 60 ∗ RAVE

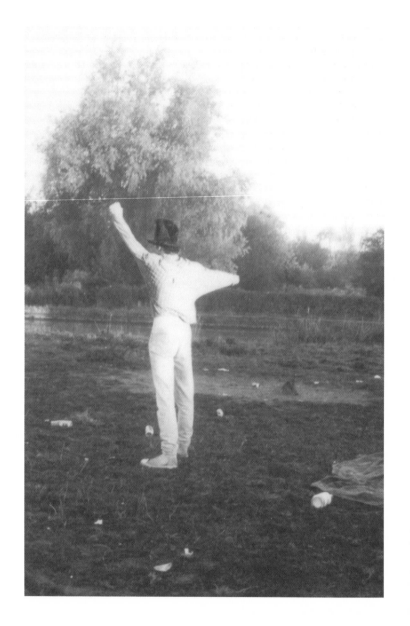

PLATE NO. 61 * RAVE

N U - R A V E — Nu-Rave ushered in the return of glow sticks and fluorescent clothing. This Acid-House-Sci-Fi-Punk scene grew out of an attempt to recycle the Eighties pop genre. Arguably it didn't exist outside of Hoxton, East London's fashion crucible – and has already disappeared. Sunday club BoomBox (set up in 2006) became *the* gay-boy, art-school, fashion-crowd Mecca (Kylie Minogue showcased her 2007 single '2 Hearts' there) and chief proponent of Nu-Rave. People dressed up. The theatrical, tranny element of BoomBox was, in many ways, a spin-off of legendary 1985–87 club Taboo, created by Leigh Bowery. At Taboo the doorman Mark held a mirror up to the queuing art and fashion students and said, 'Would *you* let yourself in?'

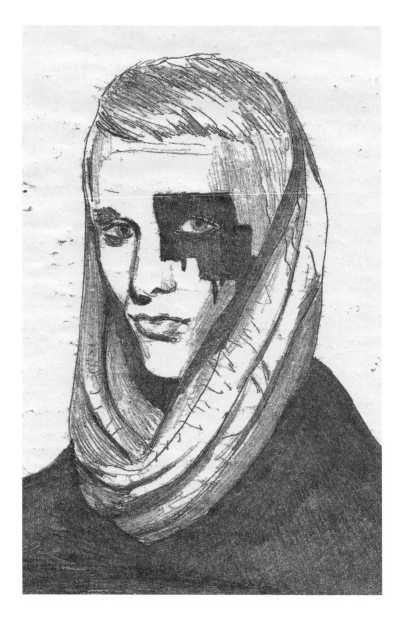

PLATE NO. 62 • NU-RAVE

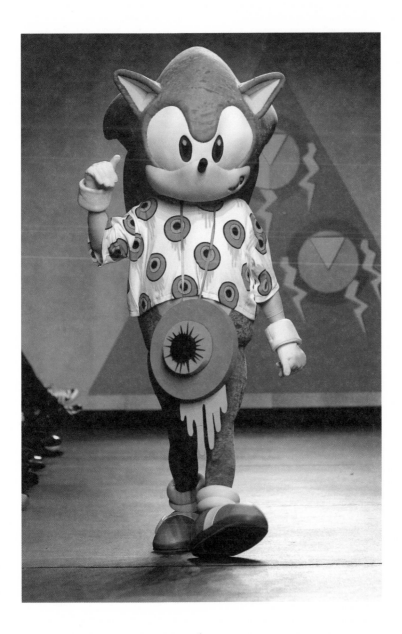

PLATE NO. 63 * NU-RAVE

HOXTONITES — Once upon a time, many moons ago, I sat in a distinctly shabby pub called the Bricklayer's Arms on Charlotte Road, East London, a pub that played a comfortable home from home to old men in varying degrees of lethargic inebriation and had a particularly characterful and enterprising landlady called Vicki. I remember thinking that I was a million miles away from civilisation and was slightly concerned about how on earth I would get home as I had never seen a black cab in the area. Since then the Bricklayer's has taken on near-mythical status.

My friend Giles moved into a disused bank in the mid-Nineties around the corner from this pub together with a bevy of mice and rabbit friends. Just previous to this, my flatmate Katie had moved her offices to a rather desolate open-plan space on Old Street with the few it took to cobble together her landmark magazine, *Dazed & Confused*. The geographical boundaries of Shoreditch seemed a bleak but rather fun landscape. At the weekend the area was completely deserted. Milk was a commodity impossible to purchase. We weren't the first to move to the area. Before us there was East End god Alexander McQueen who housed his studio there and would drink in the London Apprentice (later the 333), bought in 1990 by the aforementioned colourful Vicki.

I remember sitting on Giles's roof at the bank looking out on a rather grimy and undeveloped but bubbling industrial view when Tony Blair came into power wearing a mixture of APC, Helmut Lang and Carhartt (me, not the former prime minister).

Hoxton gathered momentum rather speedily as rejuvenation goes, prompting McQueen to chide, 'One day we looked out of the window and there were a load of people with mullets.' That's sort of how quickly it happened. The Bricklayer's was unrecognisable

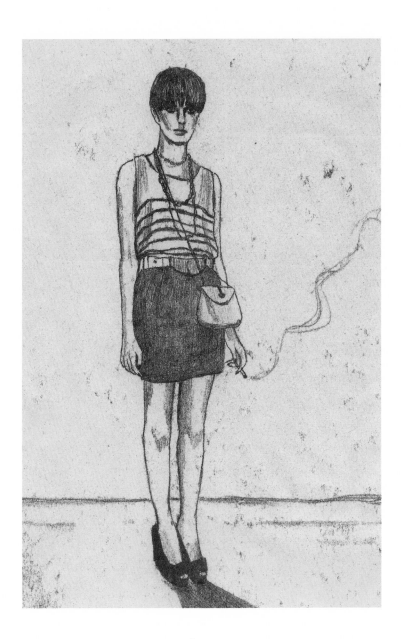

PLATE NO. 64 * HOXTONITES

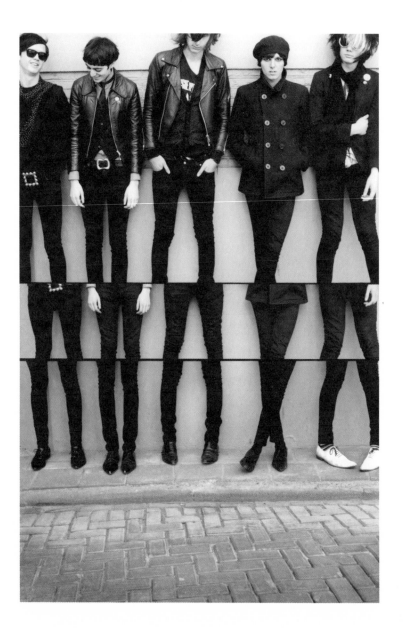

within a couple of years, but still fun for quite a while. A fellow St Martins' student, David Waddington, took it over and turned the upstairs into a restaurant before moving on to another project that was to prove rather successful – namely Bistrotheque, a restaurant in Bethnal Green. White Cube moved into Hoxton Square, which cemented the square as the home of the Brit Art movement and gazillions of galleries opened in its wake.

My friend James bought a disused school in Arnold Circus in 1999, behind Shoreditch High Street which seemed way off any safe rejuvenation territory. Its previous use had obviously been some improvised, crude brothel. With a security company that kept dogs that looked like the rabid one in *Fantastic Mr Fox* supposedly guarding the place, and a bit of whitewash, I, Giles and Steve Mackey braved the conditions and moved in with abundant trepidation and a few industrial sewing machines and mixing decks.

In what seemed like minutes, although it was, in fact, a good few years, it was possible to buy popular commodities like coffee and gentrified sandwiches without getting a bus. In later years we even had our own rather splendid canteen when the creators of St John and The French House moved in.

From the initial few comparatively inoffensive mullets, the air turned decidedly and desperately chic. An exceedingly cool and bracingly hip wind now blew through E2 and the Hoxtonian was born. To be a modern Hoxtonian meant taking a sacred and sincere oath to the gods and goddesses of self-obsessed cool – nothing would mar their devotion to the achingly sublime and they could kneel for hours with bleeding knees at the altar of cool. Nothing else mattered, literally – this was a tribe with no political battle, no real feeling or soundtrack, except being really, really fashionably brash and cliquey in their very own urban playground.

Taking their cue from the Indie androgyny of Britpop, Justine Frischmann's and Brett Anderson's hair for instance, they bred like rabbits out here. Jarvis Cocker (who owned a house in Hackney) and his merry band of *Grange Hill* lookalikes (Jarvis as the teacher, Steve Mackey and Mark Webber the pupils) inspired a kind of ironic, slightly Seventies, gangly level to the Hoxtonian. Grunge, and the skinny jeans, band T-shirts and the middle partings it left in its wake, added another part to the mixture. The early Nineties love of Carhartt, all things utility and workwear and sweatshirts bearing the images of obscure New York record labels (and the record collections to match) finished the pungent cocktail. Vintage one-upmanship became a huge status symbol within the growing group and ironic plastic hair accessories and jewellery (inspired by fluorescent beaded belts by Miss Katie Hillier) were the little iced gems on the top of the cake of the Hoxtonian.

Like downtown New York in the Eighties, this square mile of London's East End has become the sometimes brilliantly creative, sometimes desperately predictable melting pot of art and fashion. Girls in cowboy boots and X-Ray specs hang off the arms of skinny jean boys with asymmetric haircuts, John McEnroe sweatbands and retro moustaches, who resemble real-life models in one of those rather too brash and suggestive Terry Richardson American Apparel ads. Most nights they can be found drinking free beer at any one of the art openings taking place in the hundreds of East End galleries, or at the plethora of members' clubs opening by the minute as they attempt to redefine 'cool' for their generation. Of course, the real reason for the area's achingly cool factor is its diversity. Most long-term residents of the area live in the twenty or so council estates that run through it. East End mythology used to be associated with the Kray Twins in their dark suits and cigarette ties escorting metallic-haired molls to gambling clubs; now it's all about the beautiful people wearing obscure Nike trainers, watched by bemused long-term Eastenders. Most telling these days are the coach tours from Claridge's hotel to the East End, laid on for American art collectors – it's still quite a trek from W1, you know.

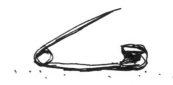

TYPICAL
ENGLISH GARB

—

THE GREATCOAT — Not just a coat but more a way of life in our nation, the greatcoat is a symbol of a slouching, hands-deep-in-pockets, withdrawn kind of an attitude. It is obligatory wearing for students everywhere, just as Graham Greene is obligatory reading and *Withnail and I* is obligatory watching. And talking of that iconic scoundrel, what Withnail did for the humble greatcoat is worthy of a fashion knighthood. Withnail wore his coat with a truly English single-mindedness, never shedding, it thanks, in part, to typical English weather and living conditions. This Harrow old boy – privileged and penniless, a thoroughly romantic English condition – lived in a squalid and freezing flat in Camden and escaped to a squalid (but posh) freezing cottage in Cumbria. His look was thus cemented in the English consciousness – a look that consisted of said coat, a huge, untucked white shirt, a waistcoat, a tie, cords and a roll-up. Sound familiar? It's a uniform – and a way of life – lovingly copied by copious numbers of students, out-of-work actors, poets, writers and anyone with a semi-flamboyant disposition living in England in the Seventies, Eighties and beyond.

There is even a cult comic devoted to the greatcoat, called *The Really Heavy Greatcoat*. It's a comic strip revolving round 'a sentient greatcoat' found in an Oxfam shop and its owner – a local council worker who wants to rediscover what pre-Thatcher students got up to. When one's mind drifts through the history of the greatcoat, who could fend off the ever-so-inspirational Fagin, Dodger and Bill Sykes from *Oliver?* If ever there's a style worth emulating it's that of the Artful Dodger – oversized greatcoat, cravat and top hat. Then came Paul Simonon in a grey army version giving the greatcoat the golden keys to the world of Punk and, with it, a more sardonic incarnation. Ian McCulloch took

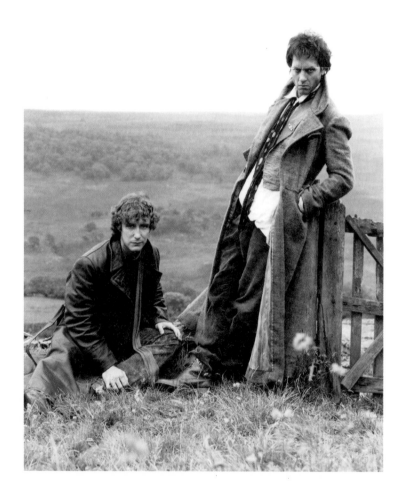

PLATE NO. 66 • THE GREATCOAT

the coat in another direction, making an image of beautiful reticence before a backdrop of the Liver Bird.

The origin of this great greatcoat comes from the army, another pattern to be found in English style, for Army & Navy – or its spirit now the last shop in the chain is gone – is style mecca for any discerning Englander. British army officers first wore greatcoats, and they were the preserve of the upper classes and the wealthy as casual wear. When the Industrial Revolution kicked in it became a staple among all social classes. It is a coat still steeped in our social structure, carrying an upper-class heritage and regularly worn by posh adolescents trying to effect a look of poverty.

THE TEA DRESS — Is there any more perfectly contrary, feminine image than Emily Lloyd in *Wish You Were Here*, riding off on her bicycle and sticking a finger up at her nemesis, with her tea dress stuffed in her knickers? Who didn't want to be the feisty 16-year-old Lynda 'up yer bum' Mansell – even though her lot was unshakeably wretched? Hers became the catch phrase for a generation of precocious Eighties girls, myself included. I think I may have even worn my dress casually tucked in my knickers for a time. I loved those dresses – and finding them in antique shops in Stratford-upon-Avon on Saturdays with my mum.

Seaside towns, first experiences of sex and tea dresses all seem strangely synergistic. The thing about tea dresses is they are really sexy, especially those Forties ones with buttons down the front and a tailored shoulder. Ultimately they are good girl dresses, but with an undertone of a girl who knows her sexual potential – one sort of *heaves* in a Forties tea dress.

Think about Jessica Lange (not strictly British but gorgeous

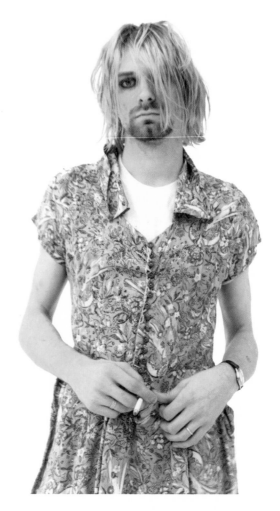

214

—

TYPICAL
ENGLISH
GARB

PLATE NO. 67 * THE TEA DRESS

nonetheless) in *The Postman Always Rings Twice* or the dresses of the working-class Liverpudlian women in Terence Davies's *Distant Voices, Still Lives,* or the aforementioned Emily Lloyd. All these images signify a feminine vulnerability and nothing does that quite like a tea dress – proper, fragile and wrongly, scruffily sexy.

The tea dress can also be frumpy, traditional, prim, Punk, Grunge – sometimes all at the same time. It is a contradictory little number, just like its ideal owner, and these complicated gems are passed down through generations, through Virginia Bates's mythological shop Virginia's (for the very posh ones) and Portobello Market, and, for the more frumpy country version, provincial charity shops.

The origin of the tea dress is typically class laden, all about social etiquette and high tea at the Ritz. It seems the tea dress (or 'tea gown' as it is referred to in 'correct' circles) started life in the nineteenth century; it had unstructured lines, was uncorseted and came in light fabrics. The originator of afternoon tea was the seventh Duchess of Bedford, a lifelong friend of Queen Victoria. Tea consisted of Darjeeling, sandwiches and cakes, and the Duchess thought her invention so innovative that she started to invite her friends and, thus, a tradition was born. But, oh, what to wear, dear lady? It was generally agreed that changing after every single meal was a little hectic, thus the tea gown was created – as it could easily do for lunch, and more intimate dinners too. If all afternoon tea did was to inspire a dress it would have been a worthy cause in itself.

Anyway, enough of origins and back to popular culture. The Sixties and Seventies gave us a nice line in tea dresses thanks to the likes of Barbara Hulanicki and Laura Ashley – the former using polyester and cat prints, the latter going floral and conjuring up images of rural Wales and ladies wearing diaphanous tea dresses, big cardies and wellies. And, pray, where would early Nineties Grunge be without the versatility of the tea dress, and its hints of vulnerability? David Sims very cleverly defined a generation when he dressed Kurt Cobain in a grubby and very English tea dress. Since then, Kate Moss has never looked back. She wore tea dresses then and she still wears them, the tea dress being an important component of her Topshop collections.

Last, but not least, the tea dress does a very clever thing when it envelops a frumpy British form. Any big-bosomed matron starts to look like a fair country maiden in the summertime, and our more androgynous, stern and skinny frumps are transformed into Virginia Woolf or Sylvia Plath (who combined hers with a cardi – tea dresses do have an incredible natural synergy with a woolly cardi and poetry/prose).

THE CAVALRY JACKET — Ever since Peter Blake came up with a catchy, clever idea for a Beatles cover with John Lennon and his band of merry, psychedelic men wearing a bevy of multi-coloured cavalry jackets, said jacket has become recognised as the national symbol of rock and roll. Sixties boutique I Was Lord Kitchener's Valet – on Portobello Road – inspired the Beatles' Sgt Pepper uniforms and the appeal of the cavalry jacket's heavy gold embellishment remains undiminished. Cavalry jackets are colourful, elegant and brilliantly tailored. They somehow make everyone look cool and handsome, turning otherwise ordinary human beings (male or female) into the likes of Sergeant Francis Troy in *Far From the Madding Crowd*. They are also durable, can handle the abuse of a rock and roll lifestyle and, once they have reached the second-hand shop, cheap.

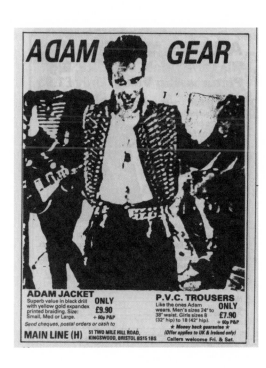

Most of our musical greats have at some point donned an incarnation of military clothing – with varying degrees of controversy – but no item is as rich as the cavalry jacket with all that gold and frogging and buttons and trim. The cavalry jacket is less about the aggression offered by the other staples of military clothing, and more about ostentatious irreverence and colour.

Okay, so an American was probably the most famous wearer of the cavalry jacket, him being the gallant Jimi Hendrix. But I would have to make a case for Adam Ant being up there as a close second – not an equal to him in guitar skills, you understand, but maybe, at a push, in terms of style. Whatever, Adam Ant was certainly the most famous cavalry-jacket-wearing-Brit and he wore that garment with a hefty dose of camp. The dandy highwayman delivered his look to the masses with flair and good humour. His very shiny, very gold cavalry jacket was usually worn with a ballooning, billowing white Regency shirt, leather trousers, cowboy boots, a stripe of white make-up across his pixie nose and beads and rags in his hair. Even without the help of Mr McLaren – who nicked his band members, dressed them in Westwood Pirate gear and called them Bow Wow Wow – Mr Ant cut a dashing figure in the New Romantic world.

Nowadays, the gilded streets of Hoxton are awash with the many incarnations of the cavalry jacket – from high street ones to second-hand finds from Beyond Retro. Owning a cavalry jacket has become a no-brainer among the style classes of fashionable London. These days even Baby Gap have a version but, of course, that's okay because it's designed by the daughter of one of the original Sgt Peppers, a beautiful circle: ancestry delivered straight to the toddler masses, heaped in grandparental nostalgia.

Note to Miss England. Can we please get some perspective on all this cavalry jacket purchasing? The best lie at the top of the Portobello Road or on Brick Lane, not in Harvey Nichols for thousands of pounds just because some French bloke gave it a few extra shoulderpads.

THE TRENCHCOAT — The trenchcoat's story involves much subterfuge and intrigue, as it includes a vicious feud that goes all the way back to before the First World War. Two royal warrant holders found themselves bitterly arguing over who invented the trenchcoat, with Aquascutum's claims dating to the 1850s while one Thomas Burberry – inventor of gabardine fabric – submitted his design for an army officer's raincoat to the War Office in 1901. By the First World War the trench had become a lighter alternative to the greatcoat for army officers. In more modern times everyone still loves a trench, from Goths to Hollywood legends and from spies to French fashion-magazine editors and artists. They are the height of chic and also the lowest epitome of the dirty-old-man mac look. But I like the trench best on a curvaceous English girl, over a pair of black tights and a kitten heel, conjuring up a look of Rita Tushingham in a Sixties kitchen-sink drama. I put it all down to epaulettes. There's something about epaulettes on a well-cut beige mac, giving an extension of the shoulder, which flatters a girl like nothing else.

THE DRAPECOAT — With a good claim to being the original, foundation-stone garment of British youth culture, the drapecoat was the pride of the Teddy Boy – 'the first mass market existentialists, anarchists and fast livers', as described by

220

PLATE NO. 69 • THE TRENCHCOAT

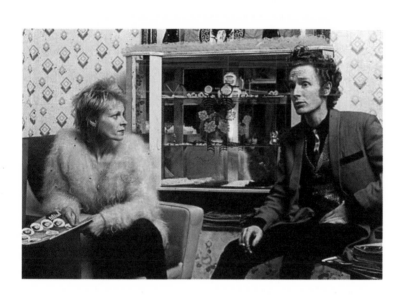

PLATE NO. 70 • THE DRAPECOAT

Chris Steele-Perkins and Richard Smith in their book *The Teds*. While America celebrated the birth of rock and roll with a black leather biker jacket, we invented the modern drapecoat.

After the Second World War, young upper-class guards officers adopted the drape out of nostalgia for Edward VII – 'Teddy' – and the grandeur he stood for. The coat then moved down the social ladder to middle-class suburbs, but by 1954 the working classes had picked it up and changed the symbolism completely, making the drape the proud emblem of sardonic youthful revolt. For a working-class man, a drapecoat announced that he refused to dress in a dull way just because he had a dull job and not much money – and drapecoats were expensive, with their owners often having to pay in weekly instalments. Where some nations use leather as a symbol of anarchy, we use Edwardian jackets or school blazers; we are not an obvious nation, it must be said, but a satirical one. Therein lies our genius. I have a long-held fondness for the drapecoat and in particular the velvet half collar, which has cropped up persistently in my collections.

THE HACKING JACKET — I think the hacking jacket might just be my favourite item of clothing in the English wardrobe. I have a lot of them in various tweeds and colours and I buy them from cheap tack shops for about £50 a pop. I like the fact that the best are not in luxury fabric but are rather scratchy at the neck (and incredibly hard wearing). But there's more to loving them than some ironic emulation and mockery of the posh *Horse and Hound* equestrian outlook and lifestyle. The hacking jacket is classically cut, beautifully tailored (even when cheap) and incredibly flattering. Somehow giving length to both body and leg, it also renders the host an eccentric, especially

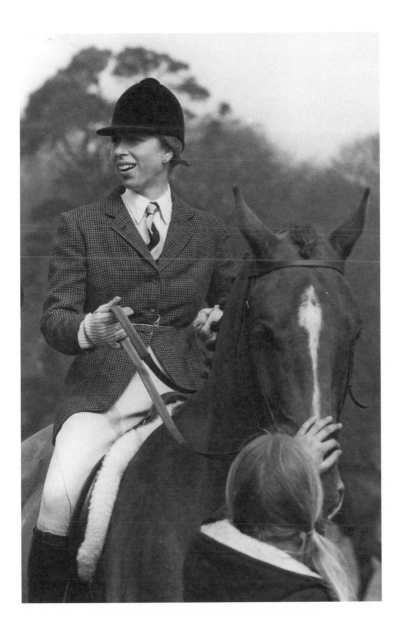

PLATE NO. 71 • THE HACKING JACKET

when worn away from the stable yard. Princess Anne wore the hacking jacket with proper grandiosity, in the proper environment and with the right accompaniments – jodhpurs, crisp white shirt and a horse; so did Amanda Harlech. I wear mine (my favourite being green herringbone) with jeans and T-shirt daily. Every designer and stylist worth their pins and bulldog clips have been inspired by this thoroughbred item and versions of it have appeared consistently in every collection I have ever designed. I am a firm believer that every girl should have at least one hacking jacket, either one customised by a designer's hand – Westwood has, of course, had lots of fun playing with the tweed hacking jacket – or as the natural, stuff-and-nonsense female equestrian would intend.

THE COCKTAIL DRESS — The cocktail dress, aka the prom dress or the ball dress (call it what you will – my dresses are a sonnet to all of these social events), gives an authority to Miss England's sexuality. I see this dress, more than any other garment, as responsible for a peculiar kind of alchemy between breadth of thought and depth of feeling.

For one of my spring/summer collections I started off looking at photographs of the last of the Debs in 1958 – these were the last Debs to curtsey in front of the Queen. That said, several broke entirely with convention, one becoming an IRA freedom fighter, another a Marxist, and another married a rock star (one did marry the Aga Khan, though). It was the end of an era, and heralded the beginning of the Sixties and the first flush of rebellion.

There is something about the cocktail dress that looks fundamentally wrong and out of place within the social establishment, perhaps a bit trashy, or dishevelled or slightly unfinished, even on

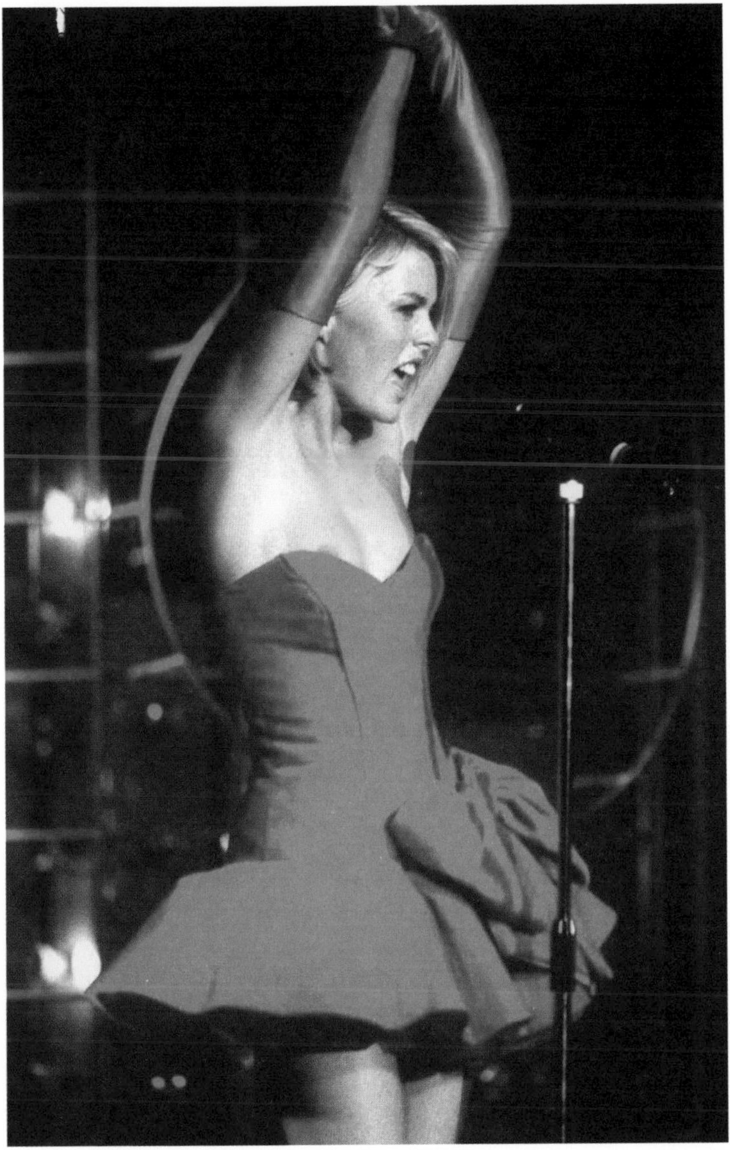

PLATE NO. 72 * THE COCKTAIL DRESS

the most refined of characters. It does not have the depth and weight of a ball gown, more her rather tarty younger sister. In a strange twist of fate I have found myself, as a diligent tomboy, inextricably linked with the cocktail dress, but for me there is always an enraged Punk undertone to its otherwise feminine portentousness.

THE BARBOUR — Practicality and irony are firmly bound together when considering the Barbour. Diehard European fashion folk may prefer the Belstaff – thanks to Mr Ghesquière's sorcery – but the English could never be traitorous to the Barbour's heritage-rich brand. Claiming to wear this most practical coat in an 'ironic' way hides, very well, the fact that many of us commoners just love imitating (with a snarl or otherwise) posh people – following a kind of Tory chic that's typically English in its contradictions. In the Eighties, the arrival of the *Sloane Ranger Handbook* – which features many Barbours – saw the middle and upper classes realise they too could be part of a cutting edge subculture (did I really say cutting edge?) and Princess Diana gave the Barbour a kind of soft focus country romance. There's been no looking back since.

The Barbour provides an oasis of farmyard style to the young urbanite, and the 'Hackney farmer' look is becoming prolific in the confines of E2. It crosses the social boundaries with relative ease, but it's a fine line, and right now it's teetering on the brink of chav respectability. Personally, I do not own a Barbour but did once have a similar-looking coat in one of my collections – the coat was entitled 'C'mon Dogs, in the Back' (I used to spend rather too long naming my clothes). I do also occasionally take a lingering glance at the Barbour-type offerings in a shop called

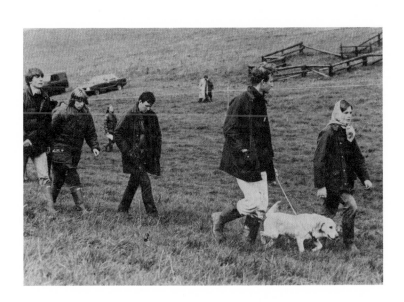

PLATE NO. 73 • THE BARBOUR

Country Squire in Wadebridge – the town nearest me in Cornwall – but as we go to press I've not yet succumbed. I did buy my dad one for Christmas, though.

THE DUFFEL COAT — Anyone ever heard of the mysterious Black Duffel Coat Gang of South London? It's a long shot, I know; they are slightly more unruly than the other great English duffel-coat-wearing icon – Paddington Bear (depending on the level of one's admiration of cute furry animals). Paddington notwithstanding the Duffel, for me, conjures up romantic images of rough but rather fey British intellectuals, invariably tutored at Cambridge, who drink strong whisky and have experienced complexions.

Weathered characters like Samuel Beckett, Alan Bennett, David Hockney and later Jarvis Cocker (Jarvis's style seems to encompass everything that was good about the Seventies BBC wardrobe) all feel like they should have worn a black or navy duffel coat; whether or not they actually did is immaterial. Certainly the English beatnik movement and the followers of Sixties trad jazz adhered to the more academic, literary image of the duffel coat.

Seventies school children also looked great in them and David Bowie cemented its status when he wore one in *The Man Who Fell To Earth*. Although it's hard to beat its original look on naval sea dogs, sublimely illustrated by Jack Hawkins in *The Cruel Sea*, worn with another extremely important item – the naval cap.

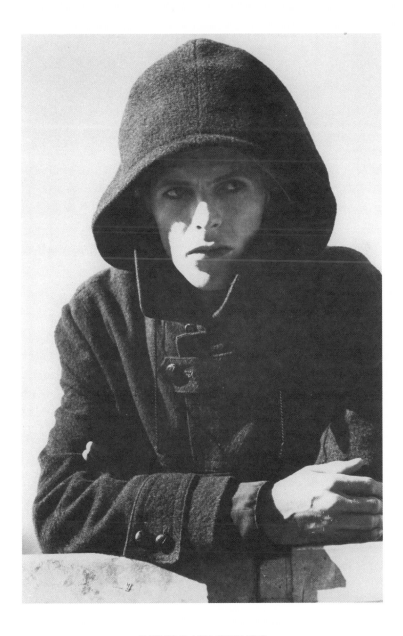

PLATE NO. 74 * THE DUFFEL COAT

THE SCHOOL BLAZER — Just what is it about the working classes ripping up a piece of traditional pomp that looks so good? Take the Kinks dressed as the Just William Fan Club or Glen Matlock of the Sex Pistols wearing a school blazer adorned with badges and safety pins and accompanied by a dishevelled bow tie. It's pure English perversity, rebellion and celebration all at the same time.

When I first started designing clothes, I appropriated my friend's little brother's school blazer and took a pattern from it. It was too small, and it restricted my arms so much I couldn't lift them without taking the whole jacket with me. The sleeves were three-quarter length and when the buttons were done up it pulled and made unsightly creases across my flattened chest. I have used this pattern, with slight comfort adjustments, ever since.

School uniforms in general have had a huge influence on my style and this is another area where the best is borrowed from the boys. What I wouldn't have done to be in a situation that got me close enough to Malcolm McDowell to borrow his uniform from the film *If.* The British school system gives us a gift of style that no other nation has – whether it's Eton tailcoats or the grey polyester from the local comp that can be so creatively customised. Aesthetically, at least, English schooling is second to none.

GREY SCHOOL TROUSERS — There was a moment in the early Nineties when I found myself going to John Lewis's schoolboy department particularly regularly, both for personal reasons and for my job as a fashion assistant. There was nowhere else to get perfectly badly cut flat-fronted trousers in the exact hue of grey. For me, grey school flannels are the precursor to the skinny jean – a bit Punk, a bit Seventies school kid, a

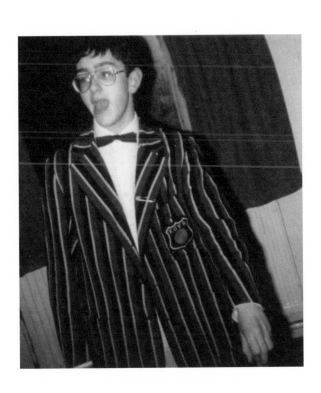

PLATE NO. 75 * THE SCHOOL BLAZER

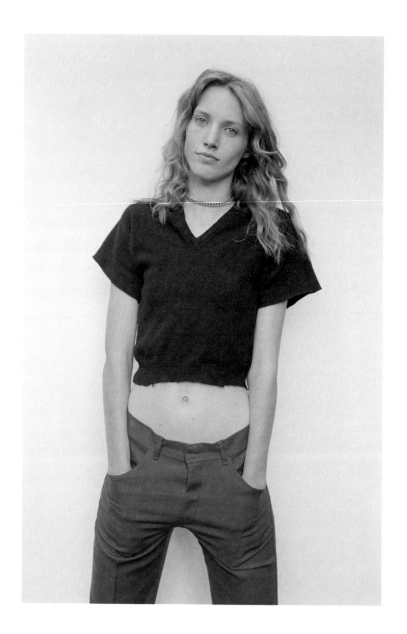

PLATE NO. 76 · GREY SCHOOL TROUSERS

bit Grunge and a bit Nineties minimal. Because they were for 11-year-old boys the fit was a bit too tight, a bit too short and very straight. They were strangely and predictably perfect, and a fraction of the price of Helmut Lang.

THE TWINSET — Twinsets make you feel prim. I've always felt very nervous in a twinset. It's like the local Conservative club has trapped you in constricting layered cashmere and is about to strangle you with a pearl choker. You can try to fight this by wearing the twinset with irony, but the twinset will not be forced into becoming a subtly subversive item for one's momentary amusement. The twinset has a political agenda and it is the most restrained double-act in the business. It has more social insecurities than Hyacinth Bucket but we love it anyway, as the national treasure that it is.

THE GRANDAD CARDIGAN — English grandads offer priceless access to the best cardigans there are. Hence the name, which can be applied to any big – preferably old – cardigan. If you can't find a grandad who will hand over a cardigan, Oxfam or Cancer Research is the best bet. Cardigans are the comfort food of clothes – they provide instant gratification, are stodgy and give you that same lethargic feeling after overindulging, which means they give the most security in cashmere (and a much needed nod to a little luxurious refinement).

When considering a grandad cardigan, the more holes the better, especially where elbows are concerned. I welcome moths into my humble cardi sanctuary – where I keep all my coveted oversized tan cardies.

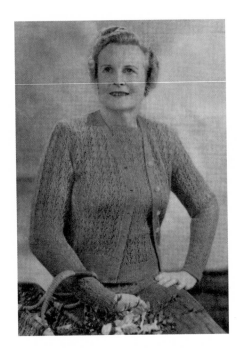

PLATE NO. 77 * THE TWINSET

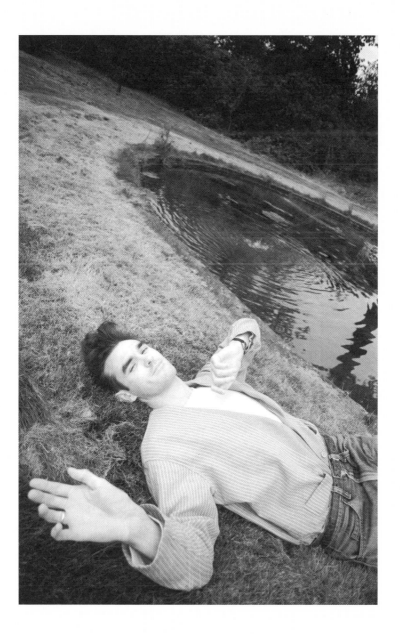

PLATE NO. 78 * THE GRANDAD CARDIGAN

THE PARKA — Katie Grand *c.* 1994, in a parka, a Helmut Lang sequinned top, an A-line APC skirt and stilettos – screaming Elastica and Hole songs with me of an evening in Soho. A vintage year for my dear friend, one of the cleverest magazine editors in fashion. Oh, and the Mods rather liked them too, fishtail ones that is, and, like the Duffel coat, school children in the Seventies, when absolutely everyone wore them at half-mast, showing off their rebellious nonchalance, laughing in the face of parents' diligent efforts to keep their shoulders protected against the elements.

THE CHECK SHIRT — A uniform has evolved round where I live that seems to inspire a sense of togetherness far more than any other item of clothing does anywhere else. The check – or plaid – shirt is worn by farm hands, Indie kids and posh people alike. Some of those farm hands and posh folk could be Indie kids too, but let's not confuse issues. The check shirt, like the Countryside Alliance, transcends class and social status and has become the national costume of Cornwall. It is also, like the cardigan, another British garment that benefits from a few flaws in the elbow area. With roots in Seattle Grunge – and worn before by Californian folk legends like Neil Young, and Crosby, Stills and Nash – the check shirt has become a modern classic, and a favourite of Indie kids both urban and rural. To date I have more check shirts than skinny jeans in my wardrobe, which is saying something.

PLATE NO. 79 * THE PARKA

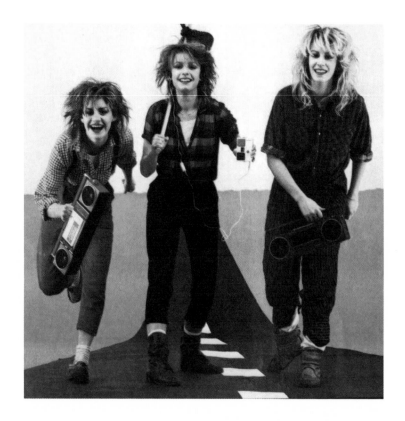

PLATE NO. 80 * THE CHECK SHIRT

SKINNY JEANS — Fashion has never been so alluring for me as when, as a 19-year-old fashion student, I saw some grimy images of Kate Moss topless, pulling funny faces with just a pair of skintight jeans and some winkle-pickers on, or Anna Cockburn's elasticated, customised T-shirts worn again with said jeans.

Since then skinny jeans have never been too far away from my persona, or my person. They are a classic, providing me with my ideal silhouette of clean lines but with something beautifully dishevelled and grungy. Unfortunately, skinny jeans are so prolific now that they have become vulnerable to the tyranny of the fashion cycle. But hey, bring on the demise. Nothing feels so good as being out of fashion and nothing feels as demoralising as being one of the masses.

OXFORD BAGS — These ultra-wide trousers were what the feckless youth of the Twenties wore (very Brideshead). Now seen as the height of English tradition, when first seen on Oxford undergraduates they symbolised exactly the opposite – rebellion, utter recklessness and disregard for the Establishment (rebellion by posh people is always uniquely entertaining, like Prince Harry wearing nail varnish). The original Oxford bags measured an awe-inspiring twenty-five inches at the knee and twenty-two inches round the bottom. The term debagging derives from Oxford bags – as a typically English practical joke consisted of tackling the owner of the bags and pulling down the dissident trousers. Oxford bags are as far from the skinny jean as you can get – but ultimately they are even more androgynous.

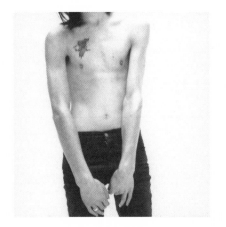

240
———
TYPICAL
ENGLISH
GARB

PLATE NO. 81 * SKINNY JEANS

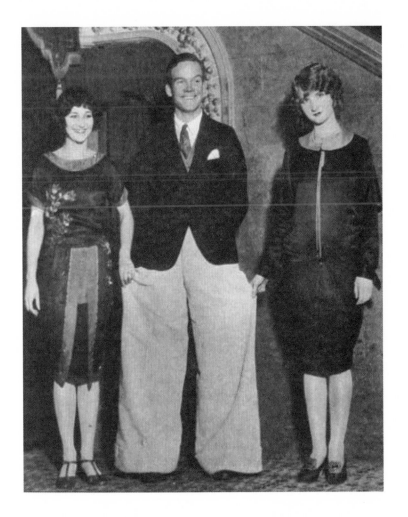

PLATE NO. 82 • OXFORD BAGS

BUS CONDUCTOR TROUSERS — Bananarama used these trousers as a way of showing their distaste of those trying to mould Bananarama's image into one that had a heavy bias on the girly. Bananarama started life as resolute tomboys with the inspiration of Punk values firmly in their make-up. 'We dressed like blokes and all our clothes were from second-hand shops. We wore bus conductor trousers that were synched at the waist,' said Sarah Dallin.

Baggy trousers, and dull grey ones in bad fabric, are a sure ticket to anti-femininity, the irony being, of course, that on Miss England they look contrarily sexy.

Bananarama had a commendable attitude towards anti-cute, using oversized men's jackets, check shirts and men's trousers to combat the girly beauty of their faces and lyrics. Yet nothing lasts, and towards the end their feather-boa'd black cocktail dresses mirrored the high camp of that particular time in the Eighties, and even their use of irony wasn't enough to sustain their original attitude. Still, their Post-Punk, tomboy moment, heavily documented by *Smash Hits*, will go down as a particularly memorable landmark in my personal style education.

BONDAGE PANTS — Yet another simple but effective shock tactic from Dame Viv and Mr McLaren. Punk has probably given the English wardrobe most of its best one-liners.

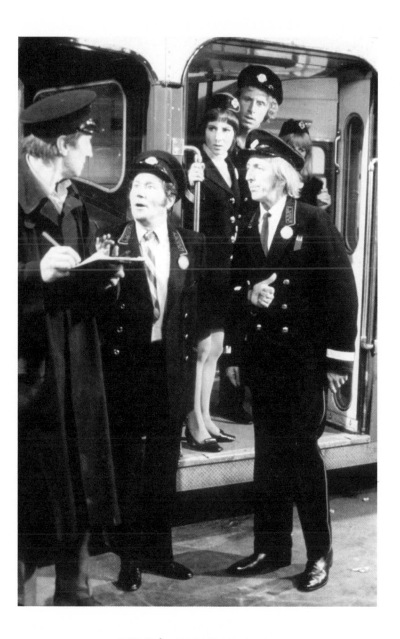

PLATE NO. 83 * BUS CONDUCTOR TROUSERS

244

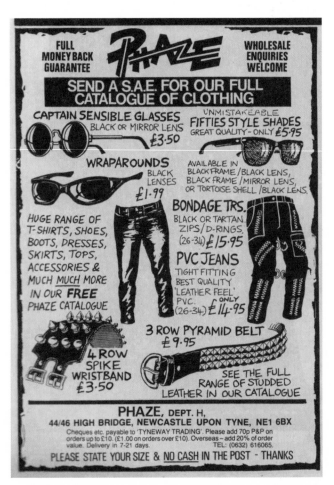

THE TOUR T-SHIRT — A tour T-shirt or band T-shirt is a very simple way of saying something you consider to be complicated about you as a person. Once upon a time you had to scour Camden or Portobello markets for the perfect tour T-shirt – or lovingly destroy the ones you genuinely bought at the gig. It could take years of soulful searching to find the right one and the hunt would become an obsession. These T-shirts were not mere pieces of clothing, they were hallowed collectors' items and worthy of glass frames – you could almost hear the wild stories of the rock and roll journey the T-shirt had made in order to be worshipped by you at its final resting place. I think the band T-shirt should be the most sentimental thing in one's wardrobe. Alas, in our times of mass individualism, even the tour T-shirt is no longer sacred. It doesn't take more than a quick trip to the good old British high street to obtain a version of a ready-distressed, aged cotton Sonic Youth – or any other very cool band – T-shirt you might fancy owning. It's just not quite challenging enough – the chase should be as thrilling as the prize.

THE KILT/TARTAN — The kilt is – like many items in this honours list – an emblem of tradition that has been subverted by those clever but naughty working-class teenagers, thus made into a sardonic icon of their preferred subculture. Tartan has royal connections but has been put, unceremoniously, through the mill – ripped, molested and safety-pinned to all kinds of undesirables, and even turned into a pair of trousers that have their roots in sadomasochism – well, really. Tartan has suffered an undignified metamorphosis but has retained an association with tradition throughout. No fabric means quite as much to both traditionalists and rebels alike – whether as a kilt or trousers.

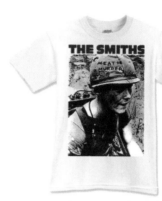

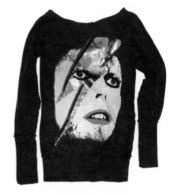

246 ——
TYPICAL
ENGLISH
GARB

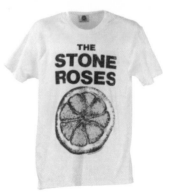

PLATE NO. 85 ◆ THE TOUR T-SHIRT

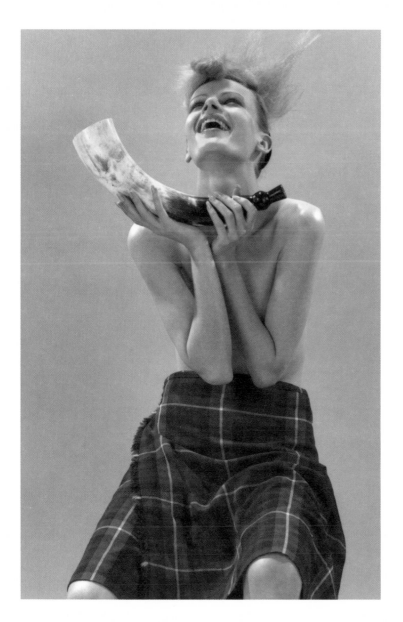

PLATE NO. 86 * THE KILT/TARTAN

THE MINISKIRT — English girls have the best legs. They may be slightly pasty, occasionally a bit scuffed and can veer a bit towards the large in the calf but this is all cause for celebration. Thus, the miniskirt is a national state of mind, whether sported by effervescent Liverpudlians or by existentialist Indie girls in Shoreditch. This was all made possible by Mary Quant, who, even if she didn't invent the damn thing, helped transform it into such a strong statement of feminism and youth that it became the political account of the Sixties. Left to Courrèges the miniskirt would have been small fry – a couture footnote. Scholars have murmured that the mini actually dates back to 5400–4700 BC, as ancient figurines wearing miniskirts have been dug up in Europe.

But back to more recent times. The mini is typically English in its contrary nature, signifying both independence and a winsome desire to please, all at the same time. It was liberation for women but also has a Lolita-esque schoolgirl quality.

The miniskirt is often referred to as the incarnation of Sixties feminism – Germaine Greer made it her uniform. Clothing is very good at stating very high-brow stuff, politically and culturally, in a simple way, in this case using nothing more complicated than a bit of seamed fabric that rested no more than four inches below the buttock.

Youthquake seems such a naff term now but the Sixties saw single young women become carefree and independent and have choices – no more slaving to be a happy housewife and only getting through it with mother's little helpers. Morality and manners must have seemed desperately old-fashioned.

Youth became a class of its own, a unified group who protested and demanded their expressions of individuality be heard. In the Sixties Miss England finally found the confidence not to dress

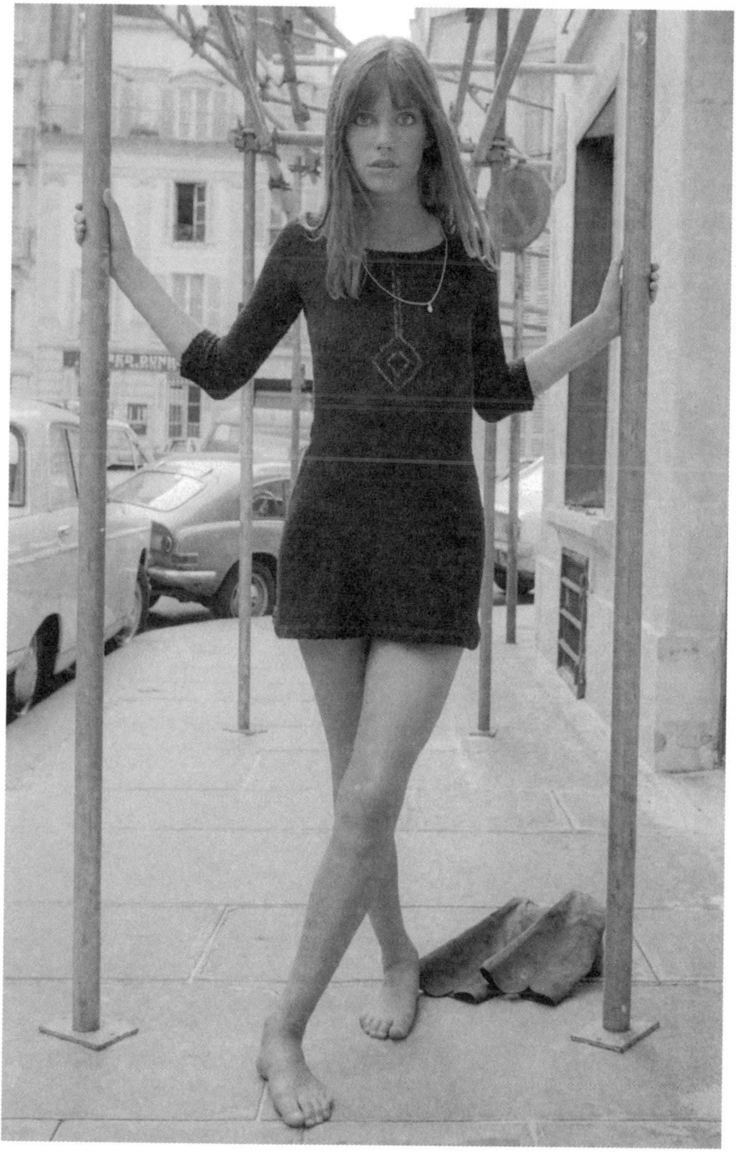

PLATE NO. 87 * THE MINISKIRT

like a mini version of her mother (paradoxically, dressing like one's mother is now rather cool and ironic but I guess that's another choice we have to thank feminism for). Mary Quant summed it all up so brilliantly and neatly in a little skirt named after her favourite car. That takes vision. She also gave a two-fingered salute to the fashion establishment, showing that style didn't have to be dictated by remote Paris fashion houses but could be every-day and accessible. But I mustn't rant about my heroine – I already did that in the Birds of Britain chapter.

But by the end of the Sixties, feminism had undergone a bit of a rethink. Maybe all that schoolgirl stuff was rather exploita-tive after all. Despondency began to loom over politics too, and thus the maxi came from nowhere and engulfed both legs and all the attention. As I said, we are a fickle lot. Punk saw the mini fight back, only now in black PVC and with ripped fishnets. And what of the Eighties mini, all red-lipped, big-shouldered, long-legged and career bound, dancing behind Robert Palmer or Bryan Ferry?

I can't stress enough how important the mini has been to our nation and to me personally. I find it very difficult to design any-thing else. Even if I start a collection off knee length, by the night before the show it has all been cut back to where it be-longs. Nothing else quite feels right. VOTES FOR WOMEN!! LEGS OUT!!

THE REGENCY SHIRT — Androgyny is a very English condition. Boys seem to enjoy dressing like girls and girls like to reciprocate. Furthermore, girls find boys with femi-nine taste extremely sexy, and boys find tomboys equally so. In-deed, this is not a modern circumstance; it's as old as England

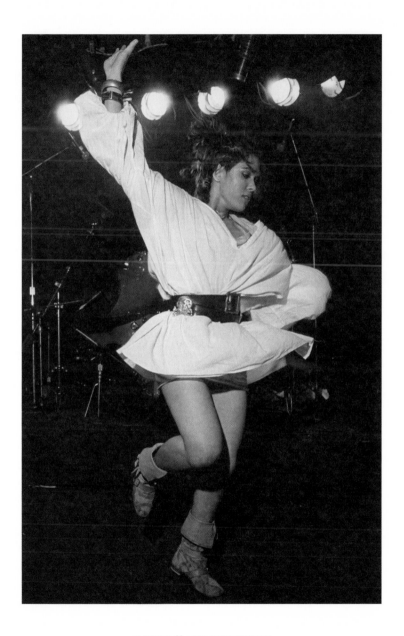

PLATE NO. 88 • THE REGENCY SHIRT

itself. No other movement adhered to this truism more than the kids of the Blitz Club, and their ambiguous, counter-sexual look was flamboyantly summed up in this billowing white shirt. The romantic Regency shirt, harking back to Byron, Shelley and co., has the same kind of lurid personality that the top hat does – theatrical and rather fey. These days the Regency shirt tends to be more coveted by girls and worn as a kind of smock, usually with some kind of swashbuckling belt and boot combo, in tribute to Annabella Lwin in her Westwood Pirate attire.

THE DONKEY JACKET — The miners made this humble wool coat a symbol of English working-class ethics and middle-class teenagers just thought it looked cool.

THE PUSSY-BOW SHIRT — If the miners had the donkey jacket to do their talking, their nemesis wore her pussy-bow shirt in answer to them. If there was ever a more middle-class item in the English wardrobe I can't think of it.

FAWN CORDS — For young fogeys and old fogeys there is something deeply and ideologically meaningful about fawn corduroy trousers. They have become the most important single element in the wardrobe of batty, posh old men from rural England who, when in town, occasionally frequent the House of Lords or the Chelsea Arts Club. The best thing about these trousers is the Cotswold shops, which you have to rummage around in to find a pair in the perfect colour.

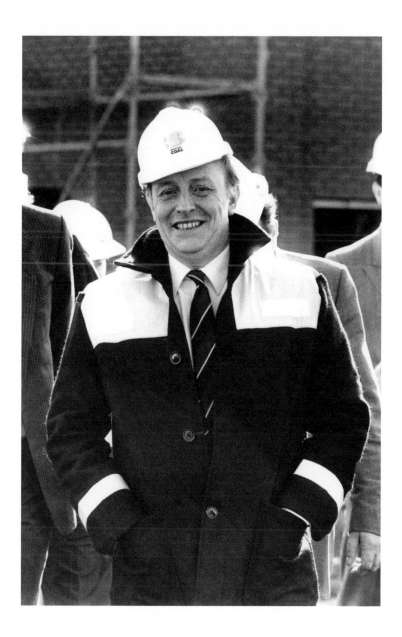

PLATE NO. 89 • THE DONKEY JACKET

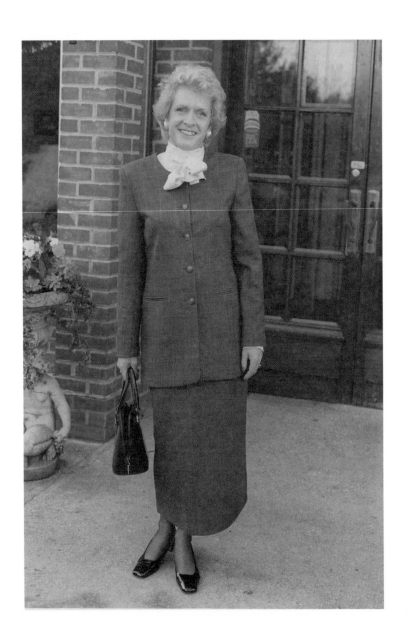

PLATE NO. 90 * THE PUSSY-BOW SHIRT

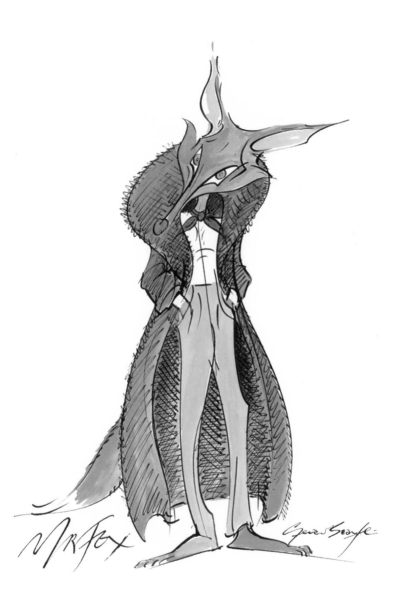

MR FOX

PLATE NO. 91 ∗ FAWN CORDS

FAIR ISLE SWEATER — Nothing projects serene images of folk and ruralness quite like a Fair Isle sweater.

It's the signature of carefree happiness in the countryside – a scene of simple beauty and innocent charm. Whether rambling at Balmoral with Prince Charles – Diana wearing hers with tan plus fours, Hunters and a cream polo neck underneath, or the fresh-faced, slightly soft-focus innocence of Linda McCartney living the dream on the Mull of Kintyre with Paul – hers adorned by blonde hair, no make-up, beautiful young kids and horses and sheep.

Although an ancient traditional craft from the Fair Isle – a tiny island between Orkney and the Shetland Islands – the Fair Isle sweater broke through into urban sophistication first with the help of Edward VIII who, when a mere prince, took a shine to the Fair Isle in tank-top form, and immediately advanced the sweater's popularity. Then in the Sixties the Fair Isle saw another boost to its status when the intelligentsia of the period took a contrary style stance to the dawning of a new era, by wearing the traditional British craft look. Pottery seemed to enjoy renewed acceptance with the art, music and literary crowd, too. The likes of David Hockey and Alan Bennett gave it an intellectual charm, while John Lennon turned the humble Fair Isle into a kind of political idyll.

THE RAH-RAH SKIRT — Is it wrong to have the rah-rah in such a discerning list as this? Oh, to the contrary. The rah-rah has more depth than one might first realise as a great symbol of British taste. When conjuring up the rah-rah, think of Clare Grogan in Altered Images, or Bananarama, or Ari Up of The Slits who all wore it in an antisexual, tomboyish manner.

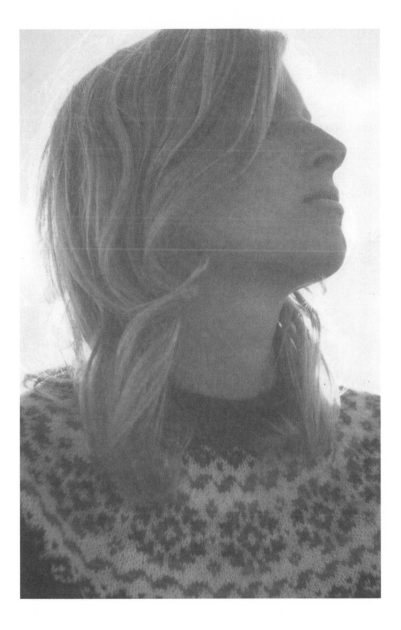

PLATE NO. 92 * FAIR ISLE SWEATER

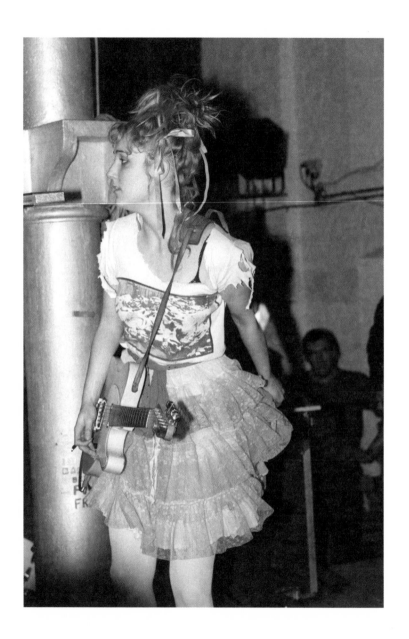

PLATE NO. 93 * THE RAH-RAH SKIRT

Clare Grogan was a style inspiration both as a singer and as Susan in the film *Gregory's Girl*. Later she went on to play Ian Beale's love interest in *EastEnders* but nothing can alter the effect she had on us young Miss Englands in the Eighties. I have loved the rah-rah since the age of ten and they feature heavily in my history.

Anna Cockburn gave her unique brand of intellectual, anti-sexy irony to the rah-rah in the Nineties, rendering it a bit tomboy, a bit proportionally odd and incredibly cool. Precisely the tribute it needed to go on to certain style domination up to the present day.

THE PIE-CRUST SHIRT — One could be forgiven for thinking that the pie-crust has much the same personality as the pussy-bow shirt. But one would be wrong. Whereas the pussy-bow shirt is deeply conformist and hard as nails, the pie-crust shirt is a slightly teasing feminine creature, especially when in delicate Victoriana lace and transparent fabrics. It is still a Sloane's special fave, but it always makes me think of a young, unmarried Lady Di with her nursery children, when everything seemed a romantic dream of beautifully lit, soft-focus femininity, and the ultimate feat of social climbing still lay ahead of her.

CRICKET AND TENNIS WHITES — Village greens and grass-court tennis tournaments – Queen's and Wimbledon – are all-white sportswear's best backdrop. The Fred Perry cable-knit tennis jumper and the oversized cricket sweater both hold a special place in Miss England's heart. As a teenager

PLATE NO. 94 * THE PIE-CRUST SHIRT

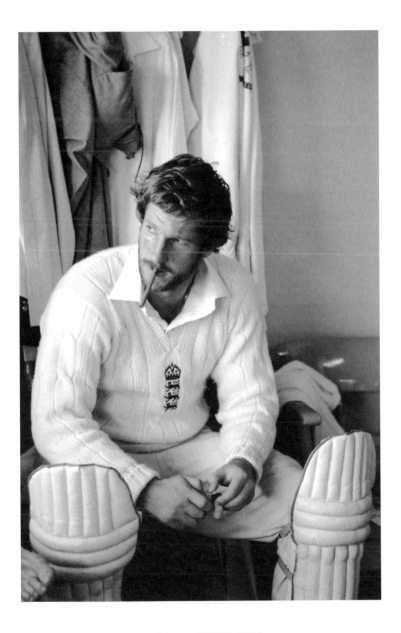

PLATE NO. 95 * CRICKET WHITES

she nicks her dad's cricket jumpers to wear over miniskirts. Then, in a proprietorial move, she nicks her boyfriend's tennis jumper.

THE FRED PERRY SHIRT — The Fred Perry shirt has a less twee disposition than the Fred Perry tennis jumper, having been appropriated by Mods, who, by sheer force of numbers, demanded more colours than the white that was then on offer. Skinheads, Northern Soul fans and football Casuals all took up the Fred Perry shirt. These tribes swore allegiance to the laurel wreath on the chest, a mark that screams of machismo and working-class heroes. Fred Perry, no stranger to the icon piece, also invented the sweatband. And he had a thing with Marlene Dietrich. I had to get that in. Although slightly random, a devilishly stylish partnership.

THE TRILBY — The trilby is an empowering piece of apparel, both for men and women, and has provided many a British icon with the icing on the proverbial cake. Ska and Buffalo have made the best use of the trilby as far as I'm concerned, The Specials looking fine in a medley of pork pies and trilbies. On the Buffalo side, the top trilby moment was when Ray Petri styled a cover for *The Face* with Felix Howard, an eight-year-old kid, wearing a trilby adorned with a feather and the word Killer – that became a defining image of the Eighties and of the birth of style magazines. (Felix went on to co-star in Madonna's 'Open Your Heart' video, in which he acted the young friend of an exotic dancer and danced in a drapecoat and trilby.)

Although everyone from David Bowie to Joe Strummer has sharpened their personal image by perching a trilby on top of

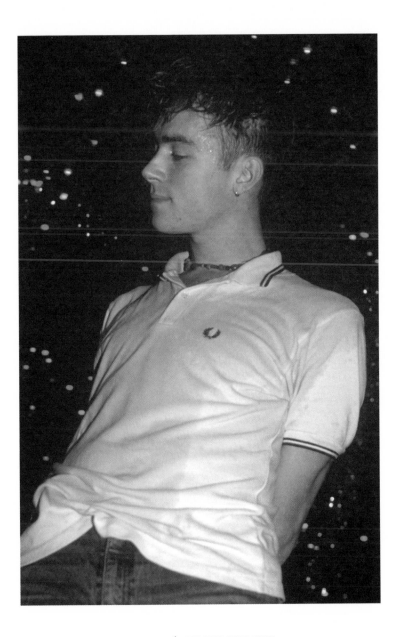

PLATE NO. 96 * THE FRED PERRY SHIRT

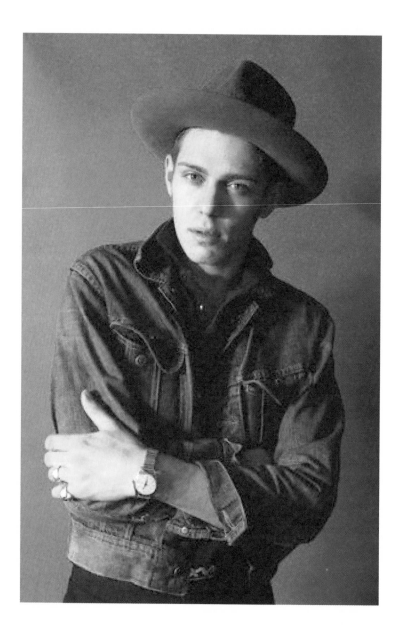

PLATE NO. 97 • THE TRILBY

their head, unfortunately, as with all timeless epitomes of cool, the trilby has long since suffered mass adoption and is now seen on LA starlets and English soap stars when frequenting rock festivals. It doesn't work for everyone. Not even the trilby can convert a bad dress, shoe and hair combo into a credible look. It needs to have synergy with the rest of the outfit to work and has to look like it genuinely sits comfortably with your story. Despite the trilby's bastardisation, one mustn't forget its power and influence on several of the best subcultures and icons Britain has had to offer.

T I G H T S — An equal and partner of the miniskirt, tights were invented specially for the mini by Madame Quant and have gone from strength to strength ever since, coming in all sorts of patterns and colours, footless or otherwise. The thickness of one's tights is now an important personality barometer, but although the intellectual thick black tight is being pummelled by the bourgeois ten denier as we go to press, opaque has certainly earned its place as a modern icon. Tights are also a political equal of the mini, as to the young women of the Sixties they signified liberation from the clutches of stockings, another enemy of feminism. More recently the rising status of tights has seen skirts deemed an unnecessary formality, with tights claiming the lower half as theirs alone. The American Edie Sedgwick was an early exponent of this idea, and it has been lovingly adopted by her young devotees.

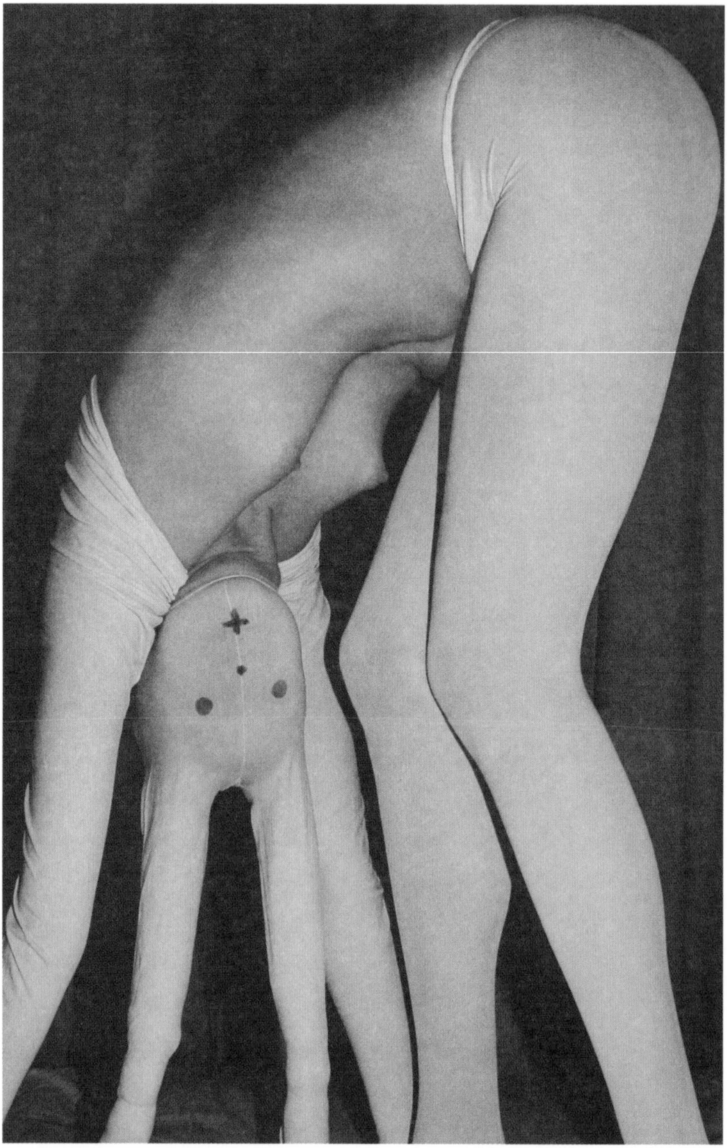

PLATE NO. 98 * TIGHTS

THE ROLEX WATCH — A man's watch on a woman's wrist – worn as an oversized bracelet – is a leftover from the Eighties, when Caroline would steal Henry's Cityboy striped shirts and Rolex. It's since become a classic for every Miss England.

THE ALICE BAND — The velvet Alice band is the stuff of Sloane legend. It's so conservative I find it gives the same feeling of unease as the twinset – one's actions seem to end up being ruled by the way one looks. Alice bands are never sexy, they are either ironically prim or eccentric, but never sexy. The Alice band in all its more hedonistic guises is as important to the Luella girl as her left foot, especially when accompanied by a bow. Hair accessories of any kind are the most underrated of all accessories. I would like here to mention the barrette, the Kirby grip and the hair bobble for their undisputed contribution to Miss England's blooming style education.

THE BOWLER HAT — Malcolm McDowell in *A Clockwork Orange* cemented the bowler hat's place as the most menacing of millinery. Even on Mr Benn it had a darker side, and when the manager of the bank punches a hole in Mr Banks's bowler in *Mary Poppins*, it's the stuff of nightmares. A deeply disturbing statement of cool depravity, the bowler was originally invented for equestrian purposes, to protect the wearer from low branches.

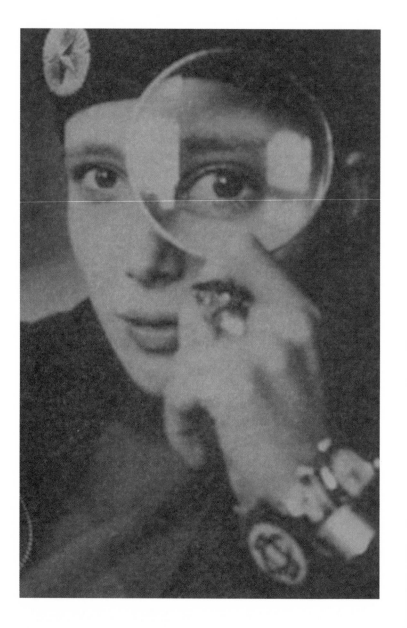

TYPICAL
ENGLISH
GARB

PLATE NO. 99 * THE ROLEX WATCH

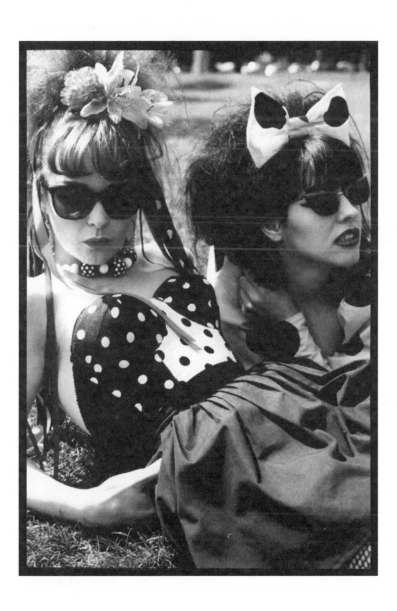

PLATE NO. 100 * THE ALICE BAND

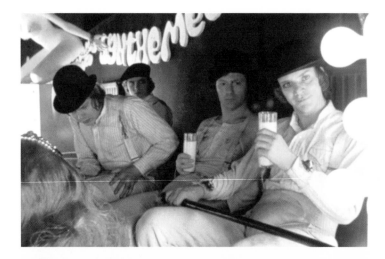

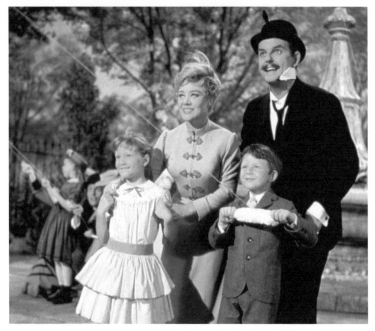

PLATE NO. 101 * THE BOWLER HAT

THE SAFETY PIN — The safety pin is no ordinary pin; this is a pin with class. This is a pin with culture, a history, an ancestry, a heritage. It is the aristocracy of fastenings. Pray, what is it about a bent pin with a guard and a spring mechanism that gives it unheard-of gravitas in the world of the British accessory? Worn by royalty (to prevent their kilts from opening up to the elements) and Punks (through their extremities and to hold together their ripped trousers), the safety pin is probably the most important piece of kit in Miss England's wardrobe. We English may have raised the pin to its pinnacle but others have acknowledged its appeal – look what Versace did for Liz Hurley's career (bit trashy, though, for genuine-safety-pin-loving Brits).

It's been said, though, that the American Punk Richard Hell started the safety pin movement, before it was quickly taken up by every Punk in England. The safety pin itself was patented in 1849 by Walter Hunt – another American – although the origins of the safety pin apparently date all the way back to Ancient Greece, when they were known as fibulae and did pretty much the same job, only more decoratively and less angrily.

There is no more signatorial image than the sight of a single silver safety pin and no one could doubt the huge part it has had to play in English popular culture. It summons up for me everything that is English. I can see the aristocratic highlands and the Punk lowlands, I can see the warped classicism of Buffalo. Ray Petri used the safety pin to lengthen shirt sleeves by ripping off the arms and then pinning them back on with safety pins. The desired effect was to have longer arms so that the shirt's cuffs would be visible at the end of a blazer's sleeves.

The safety pin is a thoroughly practical piece of technical genius. The Americans used it as just that – for joining two pieces of fabric together. The English on the other hand used it as a

272
———
TYPICAL
ENGLISH
GARB

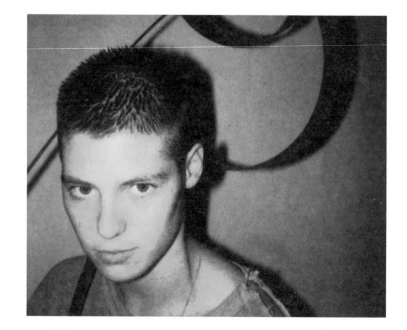

PLATE NO. 102 • THE SAFETY PIN

symbol of rebellion. The way our beloved nation has given such stylistic devotion to such a simple, mundane object is unique.

Turning mundanity into a style icon is a national pastime. One really needs to understand the art of subversion to achieve such a feat. Rendering a useful thing completely anarchic and stylish – that's what we do, that is our nation's ultimate purpose. But could there be a revolution on the way? Hanging round my neck right now is a bunny made out of a paper clip dipped in gold – made by Katie Hillier. I feel she may just be on to something big.

THE BUTTON BADGE — Starting life in the British trade unions, this tiny but very powerful accessory has since been plastered over most subcultures in British history. Punks (school blazers and biker jackets), Skinheads (denim jackets and MA1s), Mods (parka) – all have found a canvas for these little round badges, each announcing slogans and band allegiances. Out of all the great British accessories, the button badge has been the most prolific, because all subcultures start with music and all bands need a one-inch promotional circle, so their fans can present their beliefs vicariously. My favourite of all though would have to be Wolfie in *Citizen Smith* who was never seen without a Che Guevara badge pinned on the right pocket of his army surplus shirt. Along with Che, the all-time list of best button badges reads: The Smiths, Sex Pistols, 2 Tone, CND, a smiley.

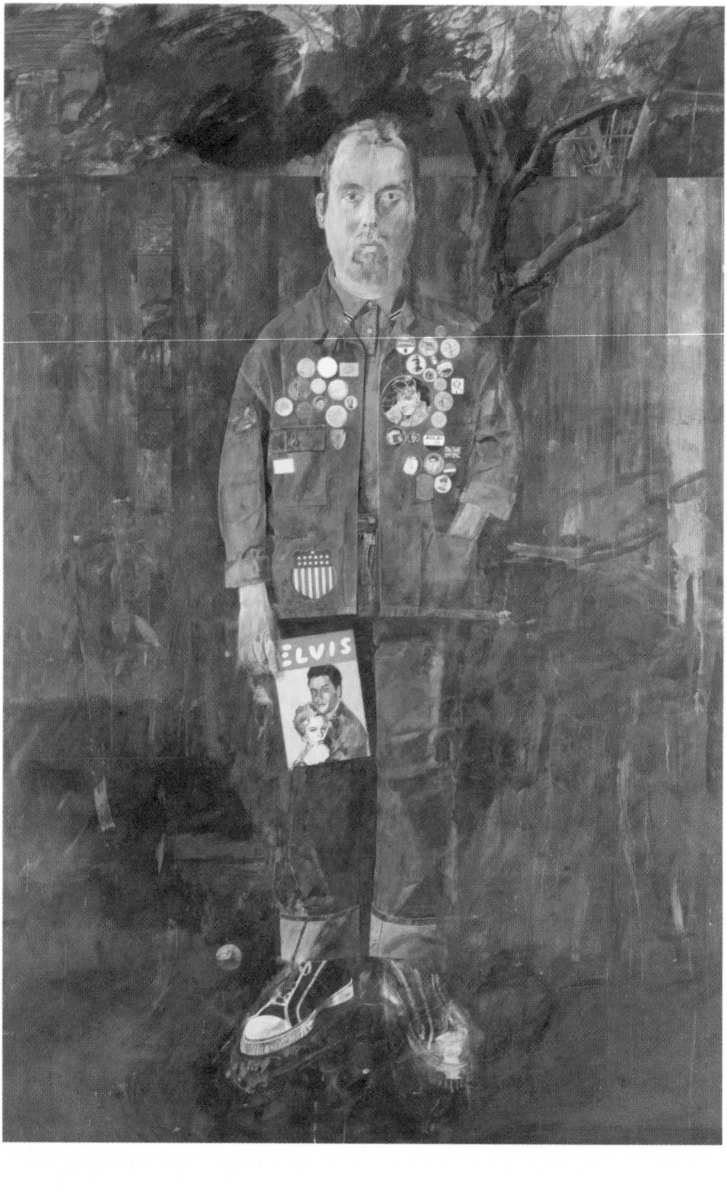

PLATE NO. 103 * THE BUTTON BADGE

THE DR MARTEN BOOT — Shane Meadows's film *This is England* – a nostalgic and tragic romp through the early Eighties – illustrated how important it was to be a part of a group, and to understand what the slightest deviation from the correct attire could do to one's place within the group. The scene in the film where he goes to buy a pair of Dr Martens with his mum is sheer poignancy, summing up the adolescent need to feel aligned to your tribe and the desperate yearning for that one item of clothing that is going to give you a sense of belonging and the confidence to know you are cool. This condensed version of the scene should fill the heart with warm nostalgia:

MUM: Wait for me, love. (He's run ahead to the shop.)
SHAUN: Those ones, the big red ones.
MUM: You can't have those, sweetheart, look at the size of them.
SHAUN: C'mon, mum, you said.
MUM: No, Shaun, they look like thug boots, they're awful, I don't like them.

IN THE SHOP
SHAUN: C'mon, where is she? (Shaun is clutching his big red boot while the shop assistant is in the storeroom.)
SHOP ASST: Now, if I can just have that for a second, love.
SHAUN: I just want to hold it, let me—
SHOP ASST: I'll just have that for a second.
SHAUN: I just wanna— (clutching big red boot very tightly). Mum, shall I just have— (Shaun gives up boot.)
SHOP ASST: Now listen, duckie love, these boots you're looking at, these come in adult sizes, you're a size four. Now, these here, have just come in from (big pause) London, are you ready for these, these are fantastic.

M U M : Look at them, Shaun, they're absolutely lovely.

S H A U N : Oh my God!

S H O P A S S T : They're nice, aren't they?

M U M : They're lovely they are, Shaun.

S H O P A S S T : Try them on, love.

S H A U N : Have they got the Dr Marten sign?

S H O P A S S T : 'Cause they're special and they're from … London, they don't have the Dr Marten sign.

S H A U N : It says Tomkins in them?

S H O P A S S T : 'Cause the ones from … London say Tomkins, everywhere else they say Dr Martens; these ones are special…

M U M : I think they're lovely actually.

S H A U N : I fuckin' want *them* (distraught and pointing to the big red ones).

M U M : Don't swear, Shaun, don't swear.

S H A U N : I want them ones.

M U M : Listen, sorry about this.

S H O P A S S T : Chicken, don't upset your mum, dear, let's try them on.

The next scene is Shaun with his brand new pair of not-quite-Dr-Marten-but-adequate monkey boots, round at the front room of one of his beloved new tribe, where a gorgeous girl shaves his head. Mum may have won momentarily, but was only delaying the inevitable. Parents, no matter how cool and rational, simply can't mess with the passion of belonging to a British tribe.

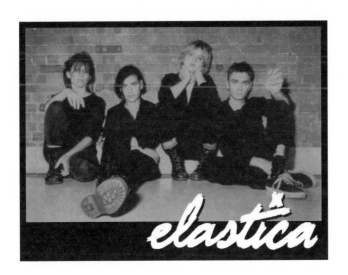

PLATE NO. 104 * THE DR MARTEN BOOT

BROGUES — A rolled-up boiler suit, white ankle socks and a pair of brogues. One of the pivotal moments in my style education. Bananarama, I will always love you. There is so much more I could say on this matter but isn't that beautiful vision a strong enough argument in itself? Oh, and the smell of a Church's brogue – does that make me slightly perverse?

BRACES — Skinheads and Cityboys alike have been triumphantly singing the praises of braces for years, never veering from their purist uniform. Both types like to put on a macho front, the former looking like cartoon versions of bulldogs, the latter like rosy-cheeked, overgrown schoolboys, and braces certainly play a part in rendering these English caricatures. Braces on girls look cute and androgynous in a comic-book way.

THE TOP HAT — Marc Bolan is the obvious protagonist of this little tale. All that luscious, freshly brushed Seventies Glam plumage tumbling from Marc's top hat couldn't be more iconic, and couldn't be further removed from the top-hat-as-symbol-of-capitalism, or the urban respectability the top hat was previously known for in English society. Since Marc Bolan's contribution to the history of rock and roll, the British use of the top hat has changed from boring and class ridden to flamboyant and dramatically opulent.

The top hat seems firmly planted in the costume cupboard and is a playful, irreverent little number that provides instant new character and gives a lot more grandiosity than the aforementioned trilby.

For me, though, the thing I love about the fantastically boastful top hat is the proportions, which give the host a kind of comic

MR. SILLY
by Roger Hargreaves

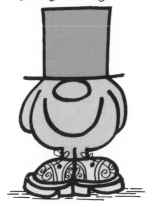

PLATE NO. 106 ∗ BRACES

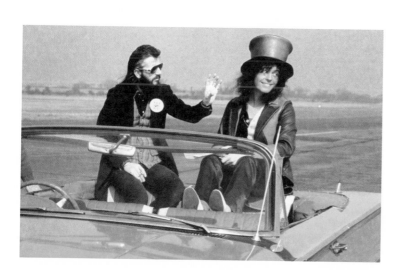

PLATE NO. 107 • THE TOP HAT

pomposity – the Cat in the Hat, the Mad Hatter and Willy Wonka all wore top hats, and people, by wearing the top hat, can achieve a similar cartoon persona. John Lydon wore a top hat and greatcoat in an interview in 1978 and affected a plummy accent intermittently throughout, rendering him a cartoon anarchist and looking uncharacteristically cute.

THE RIDING BOOT — These never go out of style. Well-made leather riding boots can last a lifetime and, in common with Miss England, look better with age. My friend Charlotte, who works at the stables where I keep my horses, had the best pair of knackered riding boots imaginable – a worn-in look that money simply can't buy. I bought a brand new pair of exactly the same boots and asked if she wanted to swap. She thought I was obviously the urban idiot with more money than sense and dutifully swapped with her condescending country smirk that I have grown to love. We were both happy customers; she had a new pair of boots, I felt genuinely dishevelled. Riding boots must fit properly for the sake of comfort and safety; I have spent more on riding boots than almost any piece of fashion.

Part of the inspiration I draw from male fashion has been channelled into my love of all things equestrian: jodhpurs, hacking jackets, the brown leather straps that I spend my life fastening and unfastening. I once met a marchioness who at the age of 85 wore jeans, a turban pinned with jewels and rode the biggest horse on the hunt; she was a daredevil and an inspiration. The great thing about riding boots, though, is you don't need a horse to have a pair. Second-hand men's are the best and can be found in charity shops on the Fulham Road.

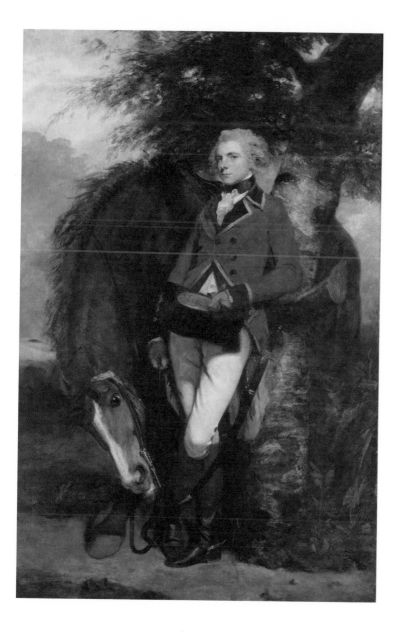

PLATE NO. 108 • THE RIDING BOOT

PEARLS — There is a photograph of a very young Marianne Faithfull in 1973; she is wearing a multi-strand pearl choker. She looks like a slightly spaced-out Alice in Wonderland who's swigged from the bottle marked 'Drink Me' and woken up in the depraved world of rock and roll. She hasn't lost her innocence or her mischievous smile. This, to me, is the beauty of pearls. They can add womanly charm to girlish insouciance – or lightness to masculine tailoring. Vita Sackville-West wore ropes of pearls with corduroy jackets and a man's trilby. Pearls can be brash *and* demure, signalling a girl's experience or innocence. They add hauteur to dishevelment and signify social class as worn by the duchess with a Dior ball dress or the theatrical monarch Queen Alexandra, who wore pearls from neck to waist. The paradox is that real pearls can look fake, while fake ones can look as good as the real thing.

Wear your pearls as often as possible. When not worn, keep them wrapped in blue paper. Once a year they should be restrung and washed with a lather of soap and water.

QUEEN MAGAZINE, 1871

FISHNETS — Fishnet tights, not to be confused with fencenet or whalenet (*much* wider), are a diamond-knit hosiery. The most commonly worn is the traditional matt black. Associations with sexual fetishism mean that fishnets *are* a dissident statement – while remaining just this side of frumpy. Would you wear fishnets to a Buckingham Palace garden party? Yes, probably, given that they now come in very respectable shades of burnt toffee and off-white. Our older English fillies consider them respectably outré.

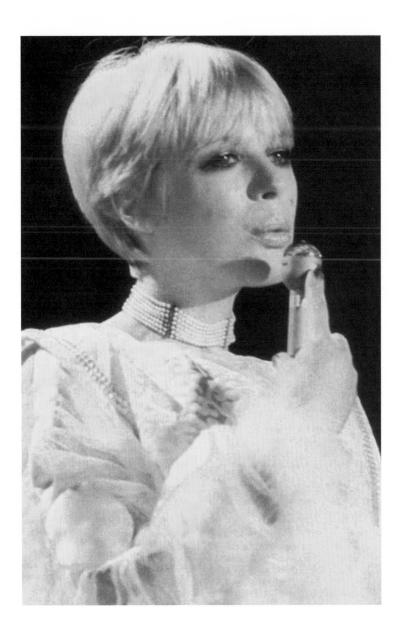

PLATE NO. 109 * PEARLS

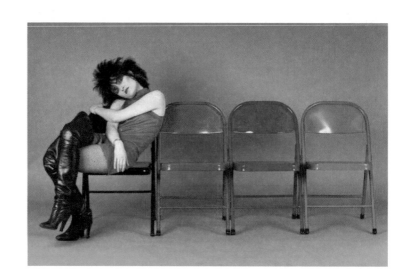

PLATE NO. 110 * FISHNETS

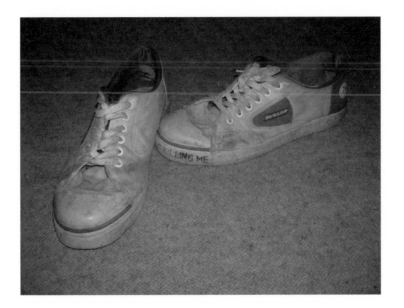

PLATE NO. III * DUNLOP GREEN FLASH

DUNLOP GREEN FLASH — The Famous of Cheltenham shop in Gloucestershire is one of those trusty, fusty old-fashioned gentlemen's outfitters, family run, where the salesmen wear tape measures around their necks. It has the hush of a library and has been there since 1886. The window displays are a celebration of Britishness: Barbour jackets, Norfolk-made suits, school uniforms and Dunlop Green Flash arranged against a Union Jack and picnic hampers, looking like a slightly deranged national party poster. The white canvas tennis shoe with the green rim around the foot is one of our classic English shoes and has been since 1870.

WELLIES — Gone are the days when the Green Welly Brigade wore green wellies. These days equestrians and land-owning types wear brands such as Muck Boots with nylon uppers and padded lining, leather and suede boots by Dubarry, black Aigles and Le Chameau (Le Chameau are the Rolls Royce of wellies and boast a double-layered neoprene lining). What you won't see them in is Nu Rave yellow or scarlet. Hunter, the manufacturer of classic tapered wellies with the much-copied side buckle, has bowed to the tyranny of fashion. First there was the Festival range featuring silver and dolphin grey. It would be fool-hardy to overemphasise the Kate Moss effect – she famously wore a pair of black Hunter's with hot pants to Glastonbury in 2005 – but the company posted a massive sales increase in the wake of Kate's endorsement. Now in collaboration with Jimmy Choo, Hunter have created a mock-croc style with a gold buckle. In a word, demoralising. I once harboured a desire to create Luellies but the aforementioned demoralisation of Hunter quickly halted the process. Still, I often think of the waste of such synergy. A welly is, after all, an integral part of the Englander's existence.

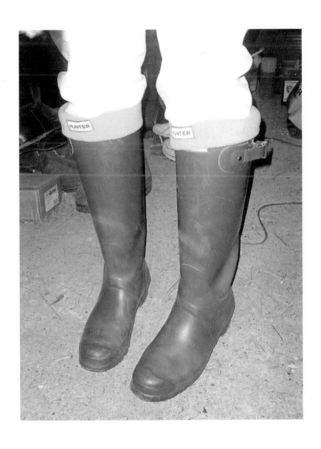

289

———

TYPICAL
ENGLISH
GARB

PRETTY
IN PINK

—

Pink drives me to distraction. The stuff of nightmares, fairy cakes and rock and roll, it sends me spinning into analytical overload. I think about pink far too frequently for a 36-year-old mother of three who wears mostly blue. I can while away pointless hours dissecting pink's wildly contrary reference points, from the fluorescent pink of graffiti to the branding of innocent little girls into Disney princesses, to the pale, posh pink of public schoolboys' blazers, to burlesque erotica, to ironic Eighties plastic hysteric glamour trash, to the seditious use of the sickest pink in Punk. Pink, it must be said, is a thoroughly English state of mind.

My design team and I used to spend days, weeks in a quandary, trying to decipher, over endless cups of tea, the social relevancy and the inherent subversive qualities of a pink cocktail dress. The end product may have still looked like a pink cocktail dress but we had heaped so many layers of contrary, dissident semantics on it and constructed such a long and convoluted character behind this poor pink dress that it became for us the ultimate rebellion. I have, in the past, created a collection from bubblegum pink, purple and orange – just those three colours. It felt like the most punk and accomplished collection we had ever done, but really it was just the most contrary.

What is it about pink that has ruled the colour charts for me, becoming the essence of what I do – and the colour of my brand? It took me a good two years to find a shade of pink with just the right balance of references, old England v Punk, and even now I'm not sure it's right.

The effect of pink is down to its ratio of red to white, yellow to purple. When, on a trip east in 1962, fashion editor Diana Vreeland pronounced, 'I adore that pink … it's the navy blue of India,' she established the supremacy of pink. In a drunken semi-existential discussion in the Colony Room with Paul Simonon a few years back, he told me that The Clash used pink equipment for one of their tours. 'Pink is the only true rock and roll colour,' he said. This was a pivotal moment for me; it gave validation to my uncertain, but adamant, position on the importance of PINK (besides being one letter away from PUNK) and why it drives such fierce political debate for Miss England. Pink, like every other aspect of British fashion, is a tribal marking; it is an indicator of who you are, where you went to school or how far you can take your irony. It is, in short, another social code.

PUNK PINK — Pink's associations with lovehearts and femininity made it ripe for Seventies sabotage. Punk as spectacle involved subverting images, styles and ideologies, usually with a heavy dose of irony. By appropriating the femininity of pink, Punks stole the right to wear pink from the Teddy boys and, before them, those Elizabethan chaps who pranced about in pink tights. Pink became a rebellious, hard-edged colour; pink became political, two-fingers up to the Establishment. Pink food-colouring was popularly used as a hair-dye. When Vivienne Westwood and Malcolm McLaren opened their 'rubber-wear for the office' shop SEX on the King's Road in 1974, the name of the shop was spelt out in large pink letters. Of course, it then became the height of subversive good taste. Post-Punk, Paula Yates matched her pink tulle and bows with grown-up attitude.

POSH PINK — 'Dear Johnny's in the pink of health.' On the other side of the social circle the pink shirt (tie/jumper/socks) is a status symbol – and the rather fey, androgynous relation of royal red. Jermyn Street is full of pink shirtisms; the Prince of Wales – and James Bond – patronise Turnbull and Asser for their silk and fine gauge cotton shirts. A certain Thomas paid homage to this thoroughly English colour by calling his shirt makers Pink – and making them accessible to a whole new demographic – namely Chingford men (Islington estate agents by day) who shop at Hackett's and like polo shirts with numbers on them.

On Fridays, the City turns pink. Pink shirts denote the onset of the weekend. On the daily commute, ruddy-faced men (self-consciously raffish, ex-public school types) in pink ties[1] sit behind their pink papers[2], pink socks visible above their polished shoes. Pink is the story of their lives; at public school the honours were 'pinks,' the colour of their rowing club[3] was pink, which entitles them to wear a highly prized pink sock. At the Old Bailey, counsel is sought from well-lunched barristers in spotty pink ties, while at weekends, our beloved English gents convene in Gloucestershire in their traditional scarlet hunting jackets ('pinks'[4]).

1 The Garrick tie is striped salmon pink and pale green.
2 Since 1893, the *Financial Times* has been printed on salmon pink paper to distinguish it from its white-paper competitors.
3 Founded in 1818, the Leander Club based in Henley-on-Thames is the oldest rowing club in England (*Leander serratus* n. – prawn).
4 The term could come from 'pink' meaning fashionable in the early nineteenth century; in addition a scarlet jacket fades to pink.

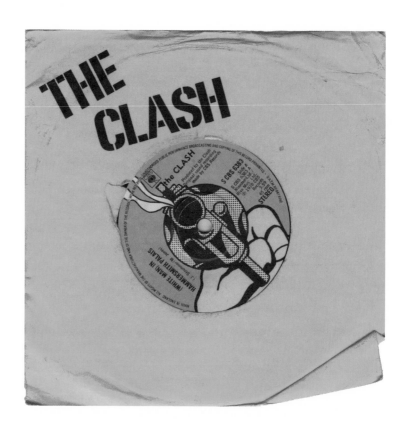

PREPPY PINK — F. Scott Fitzgerald's American Dream *c.*1927, transported to Cowes, is a world of tennis courts, cocktails at five and sailing-boat tans, worn with reassuring ease and a pink *Lacoste* short-sleeved shirt. Pink cashmere, knotted at the neck, nonchalantly thrown over the shoulders – it's a look borrowed by the urban preppy (hip-hop kids with polo-player fantasies) who offset hot-pink polo shirts with threadbare vintage selvedge denim.

PRINCESS PINK — What gets forgotten in the tyranny of saccharine pink that is foisted upon little girls from the moment they burst into the world and scream, 'Ooh, I love the midwife's candy pink cardi,' is that until the Forties, blue was considered a girl's colour. (The Virgin Mary didn't wear pink.) Pink was for boys. Pink should still be for boys. Pink looks great on boys. Maybe Miss E should take a leaf out of the boys' book and think of pink as a genderless colour, part of her androgyny. Like I said, it's all about the shade of pink.

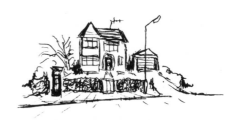

ENGLISH
CLASSES

—

From comedy and satire to academic musings and stylish mutiny, we are a realm obsessed with class – it is our warped desire (completely of our own self-flagellating volition) to subconsciously for some, consciously for others, spend our lives trying to determine where we stand in society's natural order and, even more pointlessly, trying to change the virtually unchangeable. Status in this country is traditionally non-economic, which makes it nigh-on impossible to shift one's standing within the social order, money or no money. Class is apparently non-negotiable – marriage, manners, money, houses, occupation: it seems like nothing can genuinely change your social position in these green and twisted lands. In the past it always came down to who your father was and, to a lesser extent, where you went to school and how many generations of your family were there before you. It's the oldest cliché in the book: you can't buy class.

Class seeps like an intoxicating gas through every aspect of our existence. The traditional divide may have given way to questions of taste, but how we take our tea and what newspaper/blog we like to read of a morning – every minute detail of the way we present ourselves – is under scrutiny from those we consider to be tastefully superior to ourselves.

We are all neatly compartmentalised for one reason and that is simply to give each community a feeling of smug superiority or insecure inferiority, culminating in very stylish consequences – namely, the inimitable legend that is English street style.

There are three main strands to this society – pretty basic stuff: upper, middle or lower. That's the theory anyway and complacency will lead you to be neatly squashed into your compartment for life. Depressing, isn't it?

There is one way to challenge the social order in this country. Yes, somewhat predictably, style, creativity and talent can mess with who's looking up at whom. There are the few blessed with flair and aptitude who are brave and rebellious enough to mock societal tradition and create social chaos, thus, indifferently, crashing through social boundaries and becoming the new meritocratic elite, those charismatic types for whom class matters not a jot and with whom every walk of life wants to hang out.

What lord wouldn't bow to the likes David Bowie or Vivienne Westwood (although she is a dame now; not that it means much more than a contrary giggle to her, I would imagine).

Peter Bauer (originally a penniless Hungarian immigrant who rose to the social heights of Baron Bauer), who helped to develop Thatcherism in the Eighties, stated that class is ultimately denoted by accent, clothes, education and taste. I, in my humble opinion, would simply go with clothes and taste and might then add talent and creativity.

If there is one thing the pinnacle of the class system can't look down on it's classless intellect and abandon. You see it all the time – Desmond Guinness fawning over Mick Jagger and Marianne Faithfull in some Irish castle or the tragically gone Isabella Blow finding a tortured kindred spirit in the equally tragically gone Alexander McQueen. The upper classes fall over themselves to hang out with the cool creatives and the creatives nonchalantly take them for all they've got and get drunk in their castles – everyone's happy.

Apart, that is, for those looking out from the middle. Those who try really hard to fit in, buying the right clothes and saying the right things and sending their children to the right schools, thus never fitting into anything except the group of people they are all trying to leave behind. Only the lower and upper echelons of the social scale seem to show the apathy it takes to be truly classy. Being classy is simply about lack of concern for it. The

Royal Family, for instance, care too much for status and position and wear new jeans, so ultimately come off as appearing rather middle class (this applies more to the newer generations than the likes of Prince Charles and Princess Anne, who show detached snobbery and latent carelessness in equal measure).

Anyone who actually cares whether they say napkin or serviette is bound to come off as seemingly a little bit middle class, no matter what Nancy Mitford may have decreed. Maybe it mattered once, in pre-war social rigidity, but, quite the reverse of the breaking down of the class system, snobbery has become so convoluted and contrary as to render the whole thing utterly unintelligible and even more exclusive. The minute someone decrees something as common it immediately becomes the opposite – the old salad cream and Lidl debate – the height of nonchalant good taste. Contrary folk pride themselves on using completely unacceptable words like 'toilet' for precisely that reason. It's the disregard for politeness and correct behaviour that makes someone divinely classless and classy all at the same time.

Some cynics might call it being natural, and for the lucky few who really, genuinely don't care, who are very, very few and far between, it is just that. But for the majority of cripplingly insecure class addicts, there are many states and stages of unnatural and inverted snobbery that must be treated with studied indifference before one can don the ultimate prize mask of being natural. Traditionally, this usually falls to the lower and upper rungs of the class ladder, as one community has so far to climb that they really can't be bothered and would rather mock, and the other has nowhere to climb so really can't be bothered either, and this is where they meet and become allies.

Unfortunately, the middle class apparently sums up about

ENGLISH
CLASSES

98 per cent of the country and at first glance, the middle, in stylish circles at least, is a bad, not very interesting place. Like the waiting place in Dr Seuss's *Oh, the Places You'll Go*, or waiting for personal satisfaction, waiting to be noticed, waiting for the bus, waiting for your bid to win those covetable Chanel ballet flats that might just have the power to change your social status.

The poor middle class is left yearning pathetically for acceptance by those it's trying to emulate, but can never quite get to grips with the concept of not caring, whether they are buying up titles and land or at the other extreme some rock and roll Cockney boy waiting in terror for his public school education to be unearthed and to be ceremoniously stripped of his Fred Perry laurel. George Bernard Shaw called individuals who crossed the social boundaries Upstarts and Downstarts.

One might make the easy mistake of assuming that everyone in England is simply after bettering themselves but, of course, that would be far too easy for such a contrary nation as ours that is ultimately even more obsessed with being cool than classy.

There is a plethora of the middle class (and upper come to that) that would like to unbetter themselves, trying to give the impression of a working-class background for reasons of style and credibility. Lily Allen trades off her lack of elocution, as did Damon Albarn in his tracksuit tops and fables of life in the park. Most of this downward aspiration falls to those who are looking to become musicians. Wannabe musicians make up a significant part of the population and credibility can only be truly gained from working-class routes. Recently, though, downstarting has become rather fashionable in political circles. In the latest general election the prime ministerial front-runners all played down their roots and education and wore off-the-peg suits, as if Savile Row might somehow brand them as a twit-of-the-year toff from a Monty Python sketch. Mind you, Boris Johnson has done pretty well out of that particular character.

Character is what it all boils down to. Character beats class every time. In England one can achieve anything as long as one has an extreme, unique character that is easily identifiable, be its roots in any of the social classes. Be playful, be irreverent, be conspicuous, is a useful mantra.

Contrary to popular belief, the middle can actually be quite an inspiring place – inspiring that is for its sheer inane vacuousness. If the rule of English thumb goes that one must rise from the fires of adversity to become truly innovative then middle England should be the right and true breeding ground of greatness. Case in point: one of my favourite songs was born out of middle England at its most vacant; Siouxsie Sioux's 'Hong Kong Garden' was inspired by a Chinese restaurant in Chislehurst, Kent.

The upper and lower strands of the English class system have their characters marked out from birth. Both have inbuilt marketable eccentricity – one protects tradition and the other effects change. The middle class has to create its own character to break away from the average, middling hand it has been dealt. To be in the middle is to inherit a blank canvas, to be tortured by its comfortable environment, the luxury of choice and its lack of stereotypical extreme English credentials. If the working class uses style to express its dissatisfaction with inequality, the middle class uses style to escape the boredom and the niceness.

By this token, though, maybe the most rebellious and sublimely incorrect thing to do these days is to embrace normality, twist it and turn it into the most wrong subculture yet. Or was that already done by the Sloanes (see the Tribes of Britannia chapter)? Ah, the Sloanes – a thoroughly middle-class cult, where one wore one's upper middle-class aspirations on one's Barbour sleeve – a truly rebellious state of honesty.

In truth, though, the modern role of the class system seems to exist for the sole purpose of internal national mockery. Everyone's knowledge and appetite for satire has become so sophisticated that no one really looks up to anybody any more. The intricate web of snobbery is so indecipherable that everybody looks down on everybody else for the most microscopic of taste offences. Broadly speaking, the toffs are useless, the middle classes are vulgar social climbers, the working classes are chavs.

Every individual in England can pick up on something from the next one that renders the other beneath them, be it a heel shape or the colour of their car. It's called insecurity and this is the exact thing that feeds our intrinsic creativity – the creativity that make us superior to every other nation out there. Confusing? It wouldn't be English if it wasn't.

THE ART SCHOOL CLASS — The break-off society that is art school seems to have gone some way to challenging the idea of the English class system, simply by the way it manages to jumble everyone together as equals. The art school tribe is possibly the most prolific cultural movement of all time on these hallowed shores. It has changed the landscape of English culture irrevocably and through a meeting of inspired minds plays a formative part in most English subcultures.

Art school isn't so much about learning a craft, or even being a fine artist, as finding your creative soulmates and discovering how life can be played differently and how one can construct untenable ideals that will ultimately effect world transformation, at best, or a great but rather strange style statement at the very least. Technique is all but sidelined in pursuit of collecting together a clan of like-minded individuals in order to embark on a mission of societal change. How that is done comes after countless important excursions to the pub or sitting in the canteen. Music, politics, art, film, fashion, photography – whatever your chosen medium of change, you'll find the people you need to turn your ideas into a movement. If more of our politicians did tenure at art school (there are a couple – Kim Howells who went to Hornsey College of Art and went on to be among other things the Minister for Higher Education under Tony Blair, and Nicky Gavron the ex-Deputy Mayor of London) they might understand the nation's creative drive just a little bit more – maybe a little foundation course to up the creativity level, pre Cambridge or Oxford degree in economics. Multi-media collage is powerful stuff.

Art school has churned out most of our favourite thinkers in the creative world, from Vanesssa Bell of the Bloomsbury Group to John Lennon and Mary Quant and Jarvis Cocker and

Alexander McQueen by way of Syd Barrett, Joe Strummer and Pete Townshend.

In just the same way that money cannot buy class, it is impossible to teach talent. But if you put a lot of enthusiastic creative thinkers in one place, feed, water and supply with copious amounts of interesting inspiration and teaching, greatness will grow, however it comes about. Malcolm McLaren was a typical fiery art student with more than a passing interest in Situationism. He came out of art school (St Martins, Goldsmiths and several others) with a vague idea of designing clothes but more importantly, in his own words, 'with a very – I wouldn't say clear – but a very angry and wilful desire to destroy culture'. Using bits of recycled Situationist theory, and hooking up with a talented girlfriend, Vivienne Westwood, he created an anti-culture that would blast through the political and cultural Establishment.

It happens a lot – people innocently strolling into the confines of an English art school with a few GCSEs and a desire to throw some paint around, and coming out the other side slightly shell-shocked and ready to take on and change the world by whatever means they see fit. Only as a product of art school could a working-class boy called David Jones come up with an idea for a character that would be a mixture of Sci-Fi Rock and Japanese Theatre. Ziggy Stardust was pretentious but utterly brilliant and ultimately life changing for a lot of people in England and beyond. It may start with clothes and make-up and music but it ends up as cultural, political and sexual revolution. The years at art school pretty much boil down to the creation of your own fantastical character, a highly rated commodity on our shores.

The people I met on my course and others at St Martins 15 years ago are the ones I still work with, drink with and have formed my ideas with over time. We may not have spawned Punk but there is a thread of ideas that holds us together. Some ideas have been influential, others not so much, but all have been heartfelt ideologically – even if the end product has been rather more ironic at times. Not all of my friends went on to do fashion, some went into music, graphics, writing, art direction, some even opened bars and restaurants, but the same general aesthetic and values seem to run through all their projects.

The Fifties were an important time for England and art schools. While some working-class kids created a dissident subculture, which was all about wearing your militant nature on your drapecoat sleeve, other working-class kids took to the experimental pursuit of art school.

The idea of art school was Victorian, supposedly giving the opportunity to learn a craft to those who weren't academically minded. Art school offered a release for the working-class kids of the Fifties, frequently straight out of National Service. These kids, with rebellion and a desire for a new way of thinking bubbling in their collective belly, quickly became a social type and a threat to comfortable, respectable, class-conscious society. This prompted comments from nice Fifties young middle-class professionals like, 'They wear ridiculous clothes – hardly more than sophisticated Teddy Boys.' To which the students would reply, 'We are expressing ourselves and the logical way to express ourselves is in the clothes we wear.' Ne'er a truer English word spoken.

In the Sixties new creative jobs were formed with the help of the art school graduates who created Pop Art. Artists teamed up with fashion designers to create a movement that celebrated concepts and careers that had never been celebrated before and ultimately dealt with breaking down boundaries between high and low culture.

Hairdressing, design, fashion and print led to new status for the working class, who at art school would meet like-minded people from every walk of life, both up and down the social scale. Anyone with a groundbreaking idea or something interesting to say could partake.

The non-conformist British bird Mary Quant met Alexander Plunkett-Greene at Goldsmiths. He conformed strictly to the ideal upper-class bohemian, but at art school they could meet on equal terms and his contacts, vision and confidence facilitated her radical talent. The Royal College of Art dances were the epicentre of this new social universe; the young creatives collided with each other on the dance floor, got drunk, bonded, talked and threw sparks. It wasn't just budding painters and craftsmen at art schools any more. Young creative thinkers, some into music, some into fashion, some into graphics, some into product design, all mixed and danced and created a new meritocracy that challenged the ideas of the old hierarchy.

The Hornsey College of Art sit-in of 1968, although originally prompted by the withdrawal of student union funds, became a broader fight against the Establishment and the boss class. During the Fifties, kids were just glad to be at art school with like-minded people, but the later students didn't want their art to serve the middle class. They didn't want to please art critics or have their schools run by bureaucrats. The first thing they did while engaged in the sit-in was to knock down the partition between where the teachers and the students ate. The canteen became an ideal for a classless society. Notable alumni of Hornsey are Ray Davies of The Kinks, Anish Kapoor and Allen Jones. The aforementioned Kim Howells started his political fight here, as did Tom Nairn, one of the key thinkers of the British New Left.

Since then British art schools have produced a lot of the

world's most dissident creatives who see class indifferently and have, through talent and their differing arts, created a social structure of their own. Punk was both thoroughly challenging to the class system and born out of art school. The notorious Bromley Contingent dropped out of their artistic endeavours at Ravensbourne College of Art to follow the Sex Pistols and invent the look and attitude of a generation that would become momentous. Punk was about self-affirming image and doing it yourself and Punk told you 'not to take orders from the man'. Punk, like art school, was not at all about where you came from but what you could bring to the table – nihilistic utopia with a hard, rebellious edge.

Creativity cuts through and demolishes outdated tradition by moving away from the idea of hierarchy through hereditary breeding to building new ideals through taste and talent, which, as we have seen since the Fifties, can change a whole political and societal landscape.

STREET STYLE — Pledging passionate allegiance to one particular strand of society or rejecting the prevailing norms is most successfully done by looking the part. Style is the great get-out-of-jail-free card in all the convoluted social games we constantly play without even knowing quite what the rules are, while being largely unable to explain why or how we play them.

There is one great thing about our stifling class system, which is that it inspires thought, annoyance and rebellion. The best starting point for a revolt against all the grating unfairness is to go on the attack by assembling an aggressive disrespectful outward image. The biggest difference between English fashion and that of any other country is that here the best, most interesting style comes from the street – because dressing up is the strongest weapon against dumbing down and it is the clearest and most accessible form of social commentary. In the Fifties it was called being a peacock; these days working-class youth refer to it as bling.

Street style – the force behind most English style (see the Tribes of Britannia chapter) – wouldn't have a reason to exist without the aim of fighting against entrenched elites. However, the huge irony is that in attacking elitism, our crowned heads of street style create a new kind of snobbery. We English can't help it. Snobbery comes as naturally to us as drinking tea, owning a dog and having a warped imagination. It's all rather childish really. We applaud the English outsider but really everyone wants to be accepted, adored and admired – for their superior talent and transcendent good taste – by those they admire themselves. All this is really a bit artificial, which is why we gain vast amounts of Brownie points by looking as if we haven't really even tried, while spending hours in the highly pretentious activity of trying to look natural.

English style's duel with the class system – any class system you pick, and we all have our own ones – is about fantasy and

ENGLISH
CLASSES

escapism. There's nothing more important if you think you're at the bottom of whichever heap you consider your own than showing that, actually, you're better than that, or that you just don't care. Fantasy and escapism – it's desperately important to all those who find themselves banging against the confines of their badly paid job, gloomy environment and crappy prospects. What kid doesn't want to look flash and pretend, even if just for Saturday night, that his world is more glamorous than it really is? Perversely, a warped beauty comes out of the grimness, whether that be a cramped council estate, a freezing and decrepit castle or the horrors of manicured gardens and chocolate box Britain. We didn't become the most creative country in the world simply by relying on some obvious way of doing things again and again (although a growing marked tendency to do that is fast becoming an issue for the modern Miss England – more on that later).

Boredom and adversity seem to be the best environment for style to flourish in. Out of the rain (and we have a lot of that particular commodity) comes the rainbow and out of the working-class slums of post-war Britain came an army of working-class Teddy Boy butterflies in velvet and Edwardian coats, passionately fighting against the hierarchy of the British class system and demanding to be noticed for the first time. This had never been done before. The Teddy Boys set the precedent in Britain for seditious expression against class elitism through the only tools that were available to them – clothes and music. The effort that Teddy Boys put into their defiant stance was meticulous (in England we still take the skill of mockery and sedition very, very seriously). The Teddy Boys brought sex and savvy into clothes. For the first time the kids were shouting, 'I'm as good as you', all with terrifyingly stylish swagger.

After the Teddy Boys paved the way for a new kind of stylish social dissidence – moving the goalposts of the social hierarchy around – this kind of thing quickly became a more refined art. The Mods pinched the Teddy Boys' love of rebellion, but made it all more subtle and aspirational. The Mods were the first yuppies, and though many were middle-class pretenders they expressed as much insolent aggression towards the Establishment as the Teddy Boys who preceded them. The most crucial change the Mods made, though, was that instead of settling for wearing their best clothes and transforming themselves only for one or two evenings a week, the Mod look and lifestyle was full-time. Being a Mod wasn't just something you did on a Saturday night. The Mods had a desire to blow away class boundaries and set themselves up as the new elite. Being a Mod was a commitment, and it meant working hard to afford Italian narrow-cut suits and perfect leather shoes to wear every day. The Mods dreamed of a life less ordinary, a life not dictated by the job your father did. They looked to jazz musicians and the cinema – the world was opening up with New Wave films from Jean-Luc Godard of France (*A Bout de Souffle*) and Federico Fellini from Italy (*La Dolce Vita*).

The Teddy Boys had looked to foreign lands for inspiration, taking it from cowboy films and country and western music, but the Mods took their interest in life outside England a step further. Europe seemed much more tempting than the stuffiness of English tradition and the boring Establishment, although they continued to fight against it with a passion. The Mods may have been united in the fight but – with typical English irony – they soon established a mini class system of their own. Elitism was at the core of Mod culture. There were subtle but crucial differences within the group – working-class boys were elitist towards other working-class boys who might not have been in possession of the most refined form of sartorial narrow-cut elegance. Maybe a jacket had a lower-class amount of vents or buttons, or a trouser leg veered a few millimetres beyond what was considered respectable by the ruling class of Mod culture. Snobbery may be rife between classes but the most cutting variety is always among your own ranks.

Being a hippy, for instance, was way too nice and carefree and easy and all-inclusive for the English and that's why it didn't take off as well here as it did in America, no matter how persuasive John Lennon's stylish bed-bound peace-protests were. In the end being a hippy simply didn't offer enough elitist nuance or chances for scornful aggression for British tastes. The ones who did embrace hippy culture were usually the upper classes, who opened shops in Chelsea and for whom style wasn't about aspiration and saying you're better than your background (the upper classes had very decent backgrounds already). The imprudent, let-it-all-hang-out values of hippy culture fitted perfectly with many of the posh, for whom precision, statement dressing betrayed a thoroughly unlordly approach to things. The statement of the Chelsea hippies was that of annoyingly privileged apathy.

From talking about the Chelsea Downstarts and nonchalants of the Sixties, it follows to say something about Beau Brummell. The first dandy of Regency England, he left a vast legacy to English style, which among other things consists of a kind of inverted snobbery – Brummell was the doyen of English high society 200 years ago – that holds a lot of sway now. Brummell's main point to his grand friends was that looking like you're trying too hard is naff. This meant that those who were dressing showily and beyond their means were to be cast into the style wilderness, while authentic posh people were those who dressed as if they didn't have anything at all to prove. This caused chaos. Brummell was the prime arbiter of style in London and this meant that the most expensive and grand outfits were no longer the most posh. It left the upper-class fops deeply insecure about their old-fashioned big hair and at the same time disgusted by the new modern style which meant going without scent or powder. The typically English irony was, though, that looking like you weren't trying itself took a lot of effort. Brummell said: 'The dandy is a portrait of studied carelessness but without the appearance of study.' Brummell's big idea has filtered down through the ages so that trying too hard with your clothes is still considered not posh. This means that there is a hidden snobbery among some of the more dreary posh and upper middle classes against iconic clothing, label lust and loud dressing generally – as if people should know their place. Just what the Teddy Boys and the Mods passionately and knowingly fought against.

Teddy Boys and Mods might have aped or tried to outdo the upper and middle classes with their style, but the Skinheads who blasted through after them in bleached denim and shaved heads were about distilling exactly who they already were into the most simple and powerful style. Everything was shiny and immaculate to show their aggressive pride in their proletarian values. To be a Skinhead was to proclaim that you were working class and proud of it, and aspired to nothing more and nothing less.

Then came Punk which simply preached pure unadulterated anarchy towards everyone. However, its most theatrical disdain was reserved for the Political Establishment. Punk is arguably the ultimate British tribe because of its brilliantly shrewd sarcasm, obvious contempt and witty, contrary use of British style signatures.

The Eighties brought the Casuals with their football allegiances and wedged haircuts. They started their stylish lives in Liverpool and Manchester listening to David Bowie. Like the Mods before them, they aimed to be smart, loafered and labelled Europeans. It was working-class pride and working-class aspirationalism – label awareness reached fever pitch. Liverpool and Manchester were in social and economic calamity but the kids fought back by power-shopping, reducing Armani shop assistants to confused quivering idiots. Londoners were still wearing flying jackets and donkey jackets but the northern lads espoused a more modern kind of elitism.

Mrs Thatcher came to power in 1979 and started to hone her strong ideas about – among other things – pussy-bow shirts, proper ladylike handbags and power-shouldered skirt suits. Mrs T's style was thoroughly aspirational and this, mixed with her passion for global consumerism, eventually seemed to kill off the more dissident subcultures or scattered them to hideouts in small underground clubs across the nation. The Casuals and their label lust flowered – they were aspirational, just like her – but the Sloanes, with their love of both tradition and money, came into style power alongside her and loudly proclaimed their triumph. At least one Eighties style tribe – the New Romantics – seemed to sign up fully to the more-is-more philosophy of Mrs T and its accompanying elitist agenda. Among other things this meant terrifying club door policies, enacted, shamelessly, in the name of youthful rebellion.

The legacy of the aspirational Mrs T, the preening New Romantics, the label-obsessed Casuals – and the broader sweep that youth culture was now so widespread that it was mainstream – left us obsessed with one-upmanship. What became really important towards the end of the Eighties and the beginning of the Nineties was how sharp your eye for irony was and how rare your trainers were. Oh, the lengths we would go to – pre-internet – to get the rarest of vintage Nikes. Obsessive foragers scoured the most obscure corners of New York to find the Holy Grail: the ultimate, most limited-edition pair that would bestow the lucky wearer with the smug, warm feeling of knowing they were sartorially far superior to the lowly masses who only trudge along Oxford Street and into JD Sports.

So what of today's style elite? How do we now prove our sartorial worth and how classy we are? Mr Blair's legacy of a more democratically cool Britannia has, unfortunately, brought with it unforeseen difficulties for Miss England. Perhaps Blair's ideas and ideologies were a little bit too simplistic to ever stimulate genuine cool, and the changes that have taken place under his and Mr Brown's watch have left a bit of a sinking feeling.

Global distribution has thrown Miss E, with her innate desire for rarity and exclusivity, into turmoil. Information, clothes and inevitably style are now so democratic that her natural instinct to want only the unique is almost impossible to achieve. And without being unique, how is she going to succeed in her quest for style superiority, both within her own style tribe and over rival style tribes? Doggedly hunting, customising and inventing your own has given way to browsing endlessly a twenty-four-hour instant global market flooded with generic, similarly cool-looking things which are instantly available to all. England may have its glorious history of anarchic stylishness and individuality, but these new developments are causing this historical tapestry to fray at the edges.

Now, the British streets are almost devoid of an authentic style that actually hails from and was invented there. Now, the high street is selling its own interpretation of amalgamated, economies-of-scale street style to the masses and the masses are falling for it. Oh for the days when Britain was an isolated island, free from the knowledge of where to get everything, and free from step-by-step magazine guides on how to get so-and-so's style – it was more fun. Until recently, when we had no option but to fight against and tangle playfully with tradition, class and economic restrictions, new ideas and aggressive individuality sprung up on every street corner. Now we can see, buy and know about anything at the tap of a finger and it's sent us spiralling into information overload. We can't see the wood for the trees and we can't dress ourselves with any kind of discernment. It's all too easy and the style bit of our brains has gone to mush.

The Mods single-mindedly saved for months to pay off the suit of their dreams, but now one can lazily buy into a trend with no effort and little understanding of that trend's core values. It is, of course, usually pretty hard to argue that making things easily available to all is in any way bad, but I think there's a difference when it comes to style. Can anything really hold on to its stylishness for long if it's instantly available to everyone? It used to be that wealthy women could stay stylish simply by paying high prices for clothes of which very few were made, while everyone else deployed their talent, wit and originality searching for a bargain rarity or making something themselves – so everyone had a way of owning something unique, that was theirs only (or only belonged to a select few). With the way the fashion market now works – instant imitations and huge distribution – it's harder to achieve a lasting individual style.

To show the contrast here are two examples, one from the Fifties and one from the Sixties. Mary Quant stood for youthful, accessible fashion but she sold everything from her own, independent shop, Bazaar, on the King's Road. Opened in 1955, only really ardent supporters would make the regular journey to that one store to see what Miss Quant might have made upstairs the evening before – such beautiful spontaneity – but those visitors knew that literally no one else would own the same dress. In the Sixties Barbara Hulanicki also believed in making accessible fashion for girls like her and for her friends. In some ways she showed the route to today's high street, but wit, passion and limited distribution saved Biba from becoming too mass market; her shops felt cult-like and globally significant at the same time.

When Vivienne Westwood started her label she designed and customised in collaboration with and for her peers. She priced her clothes according to their budget and consequently inspired a constantly changing uniform that, in turn, created an army of like-minded youth who influenced the world (but you could still only get it at her World's End shop or make it yourself). These days, young (and beleaguered) British design talent finds itself having to be commercially minded and quick-witted straight out of the graduation blocks with no room for rebellious playing. The new pathway for young designers is somewhat inhibiting to say the least: graduate, high street sponsorship or collaboration, meetings with buyers to discuss range plans so they, with their customers in mind, can direct your collection.

Now, our most talented young designers' dresses sell for thousands and therefore can only be afforded by a small demographic of monied, usually older women. When before did talented young British designers care for the over-forties or want to be part of the global industry? Establishment acceptance has never before been so high on the list of an English creative's priorities. Rebellion seems to be giving way to polite respectability. When again will a working-class anarchist rise up and show blood-stained knickers and a collection named Highland Rape to an audience of Establishment fashion figures without a second thought for industry reprimand? Alexander McQueen, we miss you.

All this is not the fault of the individual designer and not even of the mass market fashion industry – it's more about the way consumer culture in general has altogether taken us over and changed our world in ways that leave us bereft of some things we valued. On a more personal level, the new, all-pervading power of consumerism is in danger of pushing Miss E into unthoughtful, instant, disposable purchases. Without the difficulty factor – those hurdles to jump which make you think hard about your style – Miss E can easily become complacent. The real art now is knowing when to hold back and how to subvert the new consumerism; it's about getting back to the contrary outlook of our roots and not being tempted off the path of style enlightenment by the quick fix and the false-economy wardrobe.

We have become a nation of style archivists, ranging endlessly and mindlessly through the past, with fewer and fewer original new ideas thrown into the mix. People in positions of creative power are relying too much on the past to feed their ideas and not enough on fresh wit and creativity. The Information Age is taking away the isolation that a new idea needs to breathe and gain enough strength to stand for something, while all the instant exchange of information seems to take away the tension and force from the accidents that create English style. Again, this is a situation that Miss E can rise above, making use of her innate sense of the value of individual self-expression in order to move the cause of English style forward. Rise again, Miss E, for you are a force to be reckoned with!

TASTE AND IRONY — Irony serves a very important purpose for Miss England. She is the mistress of the craft, because of her instinctive excellence in all things cynical, but she can also hide behind it, in her comfortable, shady place of fierce self-mockery, making her beyond criticism from others.

Her diligent use of untried methods relating to her personal style journey sometimes needs a protective (and waterproof) cloak to conceal her uncharacteristically sincere passion for being competitively creative. The English use irony and self-deprecation in all guises, to guard themselves from getting injured in the action of experimentation, but also as a tool for an elaborately woven hierarchy.

We may, as a nation, live our lives strictly conforming to the values of peculiar irreverence, but that doesn't mean we want people to actually think we are silly, far from it. Caressed by the hand of wild, intellectual rebellion yes, but silly, no. If we are really honest, we have a little too much self-importance/class-motivated insecurity not to care about other people's opinions. Miss E can self-deprecate till the cows come home and happily ridicule her own silliness, as long as others can see that her particularly understated brand of inverted intelligence (silliness) is stylistically above those she is conversing with.

Really, we still care far too much for what everyone else thinks of us and if they are intimidated by our superior taste and where we sit on the social scale at any particular moment. What we are really saying when we laugh at our hare-brained and eccentric idiosyncrasies is, 'Look how way out of your sartorial league I am because I wear a headscarf with a safety pin to hold it together.' Miss E's dispassionate statement 'It's funny' would be roughly translated as, 'What a genius I am, commenting on the state of Punk rock becoming establishmentarian and what a truly inspirational work I have achieved by subverting Punk's original intention with my irreverent use of this safety pin on this iconic Hermès scarf.' It's all in our heads, you see, constantly gauging who is actually winning the silent sartorial debate of English style.

But our confidence issues can undermine us. Miss E can construct a highly crafted ensemble in the morning in all sincerity, only to step through the bedroom door and suddenly become overwhelmed with a sense of insecurity and indecision about it. When this self-doubt kicks in we neutralise the embarrassment with the irony card – 'This? I picked it up in a charity shop for 50p – funny isn't it?' (We say funny a lot.) Whether it be true or not, it is immediately an accepted part of the process, the long and arduous journey to erroneous, muddled perfection.

We treat our passion for individuality and dressing up with the same dodgy humour as we do our passion for sex, but deep down we know we are very, very good. Again, we are just scared of being judged.

The real heroic characters are the ones who can express themselves without needing the cover-up of irony, heroes like David Bowie, Morrissey, Alexander McQueen, Isabella Blow, Kate Bush. These are the real British romantics. John Lydon's quote about Punks being flowers in the rubbish wasn't a statement of irony but of romance. In the end things are so much more beguiling the less we understand them. Irony can sometimes fall prey to knowing too much and being too clever and too referential. It can be the enemy of honest self-expression. But to be truthful about one's feelings and expression can be very scary. A little pinch of irony to get us through the complicated bits seems an understandable crime for those who want to play but don't quite have the courage of the kings and queens. And irony can spawn some sincerely amazing ideas.

Through experimenting and what is technically known in the business as having a bit of a laugh, we occasionally come up with a genius piece of style commentary. There are serious ideas underlying our jests. David Sims's photograph of Kurt Cobain in a tiger suit became a defining image of the Nineties; Anna Cockburn with her version of the bumbag or the Velcro she passed on to her then employer, Jil Sander, gave the ridiculed and the bland new life. More recently, Hannah MacGibbon gave Chloé luxury irony with a ski pant; there were Giles Deacon's ingeniously immature dinosaur bags and Christopher Kane's fluoroscent pink, trashy cocktail dresses, which were contrary at its most brilliant. Marc Jacobs (American yes, but with very British taste, if not quite as obscure as in the homeland) did a take on that check bag you get in the launderette or on the trolleys of bag ladies and sold it for hefty sums through Louis Vuitton. I am not sure if this is ironic or just a very sick joke/revelation of the desperation of fashion victimhood. English irony would never succumb to quite such gimmicky irony, although the bags were still rather clever. Or did Vivienne Westwood just do a collection based on the homeless? But Dame Vivienne is, as a rule of thumb, beyond reproach.

Our humour mixed with unabated scepticism means that items at the pinnacle of undesirable can be transformed into must-have with an artful twist. The whole nation gets the joke and therefore fever pitch can be reached over a nonsensical item just for the sheer nonsensicalness of it. And because of our genuine ability to laugh at ourselves great things happen.

Beware, though, for there is a fine line between intelligent, subtle nuance and the very bad place of gimmickry. A handful of Brits have passed the point of no return with a badly judged journey into not very clever devices of debatable humour. Admittedly, on occasion I have wobbled on the tightrope of what is deemed witty. Luckily I had a team of supportive hecklers to throw the rotten tomatoes when my days doing fashion stand-up in the studio went too far. How far is too far? Looking ridiculous is not ironic and good artful irony should never have to be explained – it's just a beautiful telepathy between like minds. It is impossible to explain irony – you just know such beautiful disharmony when you see it.

The worst crime for stylish Brits to commit is a face-value joke. Wisecracks can only be administered with the utmost analytical forethought and care. Like making a rather too apparent witticism at a dinner party, your audience will quieten, the tumbleweed will roll past in slow motion and you will be revealed as the one who is inept in the delicate art of refined distinction – a horrible plight. You are as vile and obvious as your fluorescent plastic Ray-Bans.

Irony also has a very short shelf life. Once the joke is made it takes very little time for the irony to fall short. Like the poor Ray-Ban, which by foraging into its colourful Eighties archive became a victim of its own success when the joke wore thin after too many people understood it and stuck with it for too long.

Some may think that simply making a condescending comment about style is an easy route to style acceptability, but the joke must be truly original. Simply taking a luxury handbag and making it in cheap leopard-print vinyl does not constitute high intellect and concept. American Lady Ga Ga's recent attempt at irony when she scrawled Japanese writing in marker pen over her Hermès bag simply looked attention-seeking. The fact it was Japanese sent it over the edge of nonchalant rebellion and into try-hard territory.

Oscar Wilde said, 'I live in terror of not being misunderstood.'

This is the eloquent ambition of all true contrary Miss Englands. But just as Wilde's intellect was never fully honoured, humour in fashion circles is somehow seen as inferior quality. No one really listens to humorists but they can be the ones saying the most interesting things. Irony poses as frivolous but can be anything but. Bad irony is hideous but good irony is what we do best. It sums up our greatest thinking in a quippy one-liner. Other nations see our love of wrong as a sign of our silliness and our fickle nature when dealing with the serious world of style. All except the Japanese. They get it.

Queen Viv is a devoted ironist, consistently choosing erudite and conservative references and treating them with an inappropriate irreverence. She is the one woman who can preach empowerment with hobble skirts and drag-queen platforms and make it actually appear feasible.

Jane Mulvagh, who wrote *Vivienne Westwood: An Unfashionable Life*, said, 'Her clothes provide an ironic mask with which she can project many personae and behind which she can hide her vulnerabilities and even her ordinariness.'

Paradox is the essence that drives us creatively. We question why ugly can't be beautiful, finding grace in junk sometimes without any irony at all. We are simply looking at things that are ugly and strange with a different, subliminally trained eye, wearing our rose-tinted spectacles when looking at anything slightly weird. David Sims wasn't mocking the gawky young teenagers he photographed for *The Face* in the early Nineties, he was giving us a new perspective on what could be romantic and beautiful, ironic maybe, but not sarcastic. The best English irony should never be about negativity, it is more the sincere admiration of the different.

Good irony can be as simple as putting a debutante organza

dress with a Punk haircut or as complicated as the nuance involved with wearing just the right, off-shade of orange. The most refined of taste is disordered and the Nineties was a vintage decade for advancing our understanding of cultured bad taste.

The Japanese are now cultivating our ideas on oddness and hold a huge reverence for paradox and sophisticated bad taste. The Japanese revel in extreme silliness, throwing themselves into looking like a bit of a nutter, ultimately making the art of silly a highbrow, collectable art form. They love toys and plastic and will go all the way conceptually, fluent now in the subversion of their own traditions. Now, while Miss England struggles with being part of mass global consumerism, Miss Japan is hot on her heels with ambitions of stealing her individualistic crown and revelling in her point of difference.

STATUS SYMBOLS — TRIAL BY DRESS

UPPER-CLASS STYLE

In order to be posh:

1) Nothing should look new.

2) Impractical fashion victims will catch their death of cold.

3) Hand-me-downs are insured.

4) If you have to try you have lost.

5) Seasons are important: furs packed up with mothballs even if 'the season' has become naff.

6) The more lackadaisical your outlook on life and style, the more respect you gain.

7) Holes in jumpers are considered perfectly acceptable; cashmere is discretionary and scratchiness defines character.

8) What iron?

9) Tradition is all that matters.

10) The country is where it's at.

11) It is perfectly plausible to spend more on your horse's shoes than your own.

12) Cars, like carpets, need to be threadbare and in dirty colours.

LOWER-CLASS STYLE

In order to be posh:

1) One must wear one's personal wealth on one's sleeve.

2) Spend an unhealthy part of your income on one piece that gives social superiority and wear it no matter whether it is actually appropriate for the season or climate.

3) Hand-me-downs are an insult.

4) Bare legs in winter.

5) Adopt a sartorial status symbol, e.g., handbag.

6) The more meticulous you are, the more you gain.

7) The more time you take over your appearance, the more respect you will earn.

8) Subvert an upper-class status symbol and claim it for your own.

9) Change is all that matters.

10) Urbanity is where it's at.

11) It is perfectly plausible to spend more on your shoes than your rent.

12) Cars need to be pristine, hoovered regularly and in shiny bright colours.

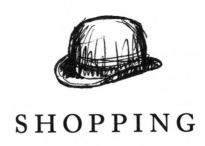

SHOPPING

———

RETRO WOMAN

Like a 3-D manifestation of the best of designer eBay, at Retro Woman you buy, sell or trade. It presents a checklist of top international designers and their second-hand wares, colour-coded and priced more than fairly according to desirability, rarity and condition; everything is further discounted monthly. In shoes alone it has Alexander McQueen, Christian Louboutin, Jimmy Choo, Jil Sander, Marc Jacobs, Marni, Stella McCartney, Yves Saint Laurent and everyone in-between. With a beady eye subtler treasures can be found: a Dolce and Gabbana patent custard yellow hairband and a skinny Celine belt with horse and trap buckle.

20 Pembridge Road, Notting Hill,
London W11 3HL
020 7565 5572
Open: 10 a.m. to 8 p.m.
seven days a week.
www.mveshops.co.uk

ANNIE'S

Overflowing baskets of lace trimmings creep out of the treasure trove interior on to the cobbled pavement of Camden Passage. Glowing bright with every tone of white, sequins glint from walls and rails. Retro to antique, Annie's is the vintage store you dream of (you and a plethora of high-profile fanatics). Flapper feels like the focus, from nighties to wedding dresses, but other pieces are introduced: fur from every era in very fine condition, or Forties tea dresses and Fifties swimwear and rompers for summer. Lace is a recurrent theme, with hand-worked table linen, exquisite scarves, delicate Victorian blouses and a grand choice of capes and boleros, mostly white to match the odd bowler and top hat in the same tone. It is giddyingly feminine, terribly theatrical, and inspiringly so.

12 Camden Passage, Islington,
London N1 8ED
020 7359 0796 / 07968 037993
Open: 11 a.m. to 6 p.m.
seven days a week.
www.anniesvintageclothing.co.uk

DOVER STREET MARKET

A market by nature though, in fact, it is impossible to imagine somewhere that less resembles one. 'I want to create a kind of market where various creators from various fields gather together and encounter each other in an ongoing atmosphere of beautiful chaos: the mixing up and coming together of different kindred souls who all share a strong personal vision,' says director of DSM and Comme des Garcons, Rei Kawakubo. Acting almost as a Comme des Garçons' flagship, it presents all the collections bearing the Comme name. Own-brand products sit comfortably beside the most adventurous buys from the best current designer collections in a store that caters for all luxury necessities.

Youthful casuals are housed on the lower ground floor beside a pocket of space dedicated to vintage books, magazines and papers. This shop within a shop is IDEA Books, the invention of book collectors Angela Hill and David Owen. Alongside often previously unseen books, finds include David Bailey and David Litchfield's *Ritz* newspaper. All offers are well preserved and beautifully presented. Unconventional chandeliers dripping with crystals light the ground floor, illuminating the jewellery among other accessories, small leather goods, scent, specs and so on. A fiercely modern interior greets you on the

first floor, as does a slapped-together clapboard hut or stockroom. A second-floor garden grows among skeleton rooms (rooms constructed without walls that you duck and swerve between). The third floor sees a rainbow of clashing Lanvin and imported vintage from renowned LA outlet Decades against a backdrop of contradictions: heavy velvet curtains meet Givenchy stripes meet leopard print Giambattista Valli meet Erdem florals growing from a steel tile floor. What aesthetically on paper couldn't possibly work, here is synergetic. Dressing room meets kitchen up on the fourth floor. Although Rose Bakery began life in residential Paris, she is English and the menu of tea, cakes and light savouries is ever so. Rose reminds you that DSM resides in the English capital, easy to forget amid the myriad of international brands.

17–18 Dover Street,
London W1S 4LT
020 7518 0680
Open: 11 a.m. to 6.30 p.m.
Monday to Wednesday;
11 a.m. to 7 p.m.
Thursday to Saturday.
www.doverstreetmarket.com

THE VINTAGE
ACADEME

Presented like the finest fashion boutique, The Vintage Academe sends sourcers globewide to acquire specific pieces to complete their meticulously devised collections. Selling twentieth-century women's fashion and haute couture and namedropping the best: Chloé through Thierry Mugler, Alaïa, Hervé Léger to Chanel and Yves Saint Laurent. Find the edited wares online, in Browns and One.Two.Five Presents. In each Academe there are no tightly packed rails, but rather a perfectly conceived capsule collection, which evolves seasonally and is specific to each store. Beautifully designed swing tags helpfully describe designer and era but do reveal investment high prices. The Academe has been branded bravely; it is chic, contemporary and utterly unstuffy. The website, along with its online store, has expert articles and high fashion editorial and there is a blog to keep you informed on everything Academe.

Browns,
24–27 South Molton Street, London
W1K 5RD
6c Sloane Street, Belgravia,
London SW1X 9LE

One.Two.Five Presents,
125 Ledbury Road, Notting Hill,
London W11 2AQ
07786 748 214 for private
viewings or more information
about 'Salon' events.
www.vintageacademe.com

BROGUES FROM
JERMYN STREET

Trickers at 67 Jermyn Street makes a slightly heavier, clumpy brogue; boot versions are available too and there is a deep tread country option. It offers a handmade bespoke service alongside its comprehensive selection of classic styles for immediate wear.

67 Jermyn Street, St James's,
London SW1Y 6NY
020 7930 6395
Open: 9.30 a.m. to 6 p.m.
Monday to Friday;
9.30 a.m. to 5.30 p.m. Saturday.
www.trickers.com

Number 83 sees the oldest remaining handmade bespoke bootmakers in London. Henry Maxwell still makes boots and shoes on site in Jermyn Street and the heady smells of new leather drift through from the workshop to the heavy wood-panelled and traditionally dimly lit interior of the shop front. Originally a spurmaker; you can see the collection in store. Henry Maxwell thrived on the use of the horse for battle, ceremony, hunting, sport and personal transport, supplying boots for cavalry regiments, hunting and polo. It now repairs and refurbishes footwear and other quality leather goods but continues to have a strong following for its ready-to-wear English shoes and luggage.

83 Jermyn Street, St James's,
London SW1Y 6JD
020 7930 5385
Open: 10 a.m to 6 p.m.
Monday to Saturday.
www.henrymaxwell.com

Church's, at 108 to 110, has, unlike Henry Maxwell, had somewhat of a makeover. Very much presenting the same formula as its extensive list of other outlets, Church's has become a favourite of the British high street and therefore unfortunately feels slightly less genuine than the dark, faded interiors of its Jermyn Street counterparts. However, the product is ever reliable and what it lacks in interior integrity it makes up for in its less stuffy attitude. It does an unrivalled ladies' brogue, just enough sole, just the right width, and introduced seasonal colours for the more adventurous.

108–110 Jermyn Street, St James's,
London SW1Y 6EE
020 7930 8210
Open: 10 a.m. to 6.30 p.m.
Monday to Friday;
10 a.m. to 6 p.m. Saturday;
11 a.m. to 5 p.m. Sunday.
www.church-footwear.com

LOCK & CO. HATTERS

Established in 1676 to wait upon the Court at St James's, the business now serves customers from all corners of the earth; its survival is the consequence of their unequalled quality and personal service. The Coke, or more commonly, the Bowler (after the makers of the original prototype), was created at James Lock in 1850 for a William Coke, intended to protect the heads of gamekeepers from overhanging tree branches, fitting close to the head so as not to blow off. Coke personally tested the design by jumping on it; it withstood his weight, and so he bought it. Today you can, of course, commission the above in black, brown or grey alongside all the styles you might expect: proper stiff straw boaters, the most finely woven panamas, tweed flat caps for the country and handmade velvet-covered riding hats. The Voyager is a modern sort of trilby, lightweight, soft, foldable travel felt for a lower maintenance hat wearer. Upstairs sees the women's department and a lot of wide brims and plenty of wedding offerings. Downstairs again and piles of dusty antique satin top hats and old boxes tell again of Lock & Co.'s history.

6 St James's Street, St James's,
London SW1A 1EF
020 7930 8874
Open: 9 a.m. to 5.30 p.m.
Monday to Friday;
9.30 a.m. to 5 p.m. Saturday.
www.lockhatters.co.uk

D . R . HARRIS

A chemist and perfumers for over 200 years, D. R. Harris still produces most products by traditional methods, handmade and packed on the premises. You could be stepping back in time from the chime of the bell on the door, to the deep dyed red and gold thick pile carpets and darkest mahogany glassfronted cabinets, to the ladies behind the counter in their starched white aprons. Packaging remains beautifully unchanged, so much so you'd have it on show. Recognisable no-nonsense

smells feel natural and healthy like cucumber and rose moisturiser and lavender water. There is soap on a rope, silky or soft bath, Mason Pearson hairbrushes, hard, medium or soft bone toothbrushes and every other bathroom accessory, both necessary and luxuriously indulgent.

29 St James's Street, St James's,
London SW1A 1HB
020 7930 3915
Open: 8.30 a.m, to 6 p.m.
Monday to Friday;
9.30 a.m. to 5 p.m. Saturday.
www.drharris.co.uk

TURNBULL & ASSER

Shirtmakers by appointment to HRH the Prince of Wales. Turnbull & Asser is classically, distinctively English and goes to a whole new level of personal service. It has been measuring and making bespoke shirts since 1885 and has served leading British figures from the famous – the Prince of Wales and Sir Winston Churchill – to the fictional – James Bond. The Jermyn Street store proudly offers the intimacy and aesthetic of an exclusive members' club. The epitome of luxury men's outfitter (though it does now have a few women's offerings), it provides all a gentleman might need for one's terribly elegant lifestyle. The gentleman shopper can choose any collar and cuff combination from a glass cabinet displaying all the options, pressed, folded and cuff-linked. Shirts aside you can dress head to toe in Turnbull & Asser, including pressed striped boxers and nightshirts with mother-of-pearl buttons and dotty silk dressing gowns and robes. For made-to-measure suits, customers can browse fabric books with expert clothiers and be guided through style, colour and fit to their liking. There are also evening and smoking jackets, velvet with paisley silk lining and frogging. Not forgetting the obligatory (in all the brightest rainbow tones) ties, hankies, scarves, socks, cufflinks, gloves, belts, braces and brollies.

71 and 72 Jermyn Street,
London SW1Y 6PF
020 7808 3000
Open: 9 a.m. to 6 p.m. Monday to
Friday; 9.30 a.m. to 6 p.m. Saturday.
www.turnbullandasser.com

M.GOLDSTEIN

The bleached, coiffed and always immaculately presented Pippa Brooks, shop girl at M.Goldstein, is no amateur assistant. Performances at Kinky Gerlinky led to others and one night, over her lip-syncing act, she met Max Karie. He got her a job in a store selling Galliano's graduate collection and there they began plotting their own shop. This led to blagging a corner of Bar Italia's launderette to sell from before moving to a Brewer Street basement and then finally to the Shop at Maison Bertaux where Pippa was Madame. Lately she has partnered up with Stevie Stewart of Nineties label BodyMap to recycle their respective fabric archives into the form of Victoriana, tight tweed suits, lingerie and BodyMap recycled knitwear. 'There's a certain old-school lesbian chic creeping in there, which I love,' says Pippa. The collection can soon be viewed at M.Goldstein, which she shares with squeeze and father of her twins, Nathaniel Lee Jones (who was/is a well-known face on the antique, flea market and street market scene). Nathaniel fills the petite space with a magpie's nest of curiosities. Junk cum vintage cum antique store, M.Goldstein is a shop/showroom/installation/idea/work-in-progress. From week to week it may change beyond recognition and this certainly is where its charm lies. Invest in the unique concept and sign up for e-mail updates where new arrivals, deliveries and thoughts will arrive to your inbox. On my last visit stock included Fifties brogues, old shop interior, peculiar ceramics, vintage long johns and Russian army Breton-style tops with a somewhat authentic papery feel. M.Goldstein with its original signage but newly candy painted exterior is a place to be surprised and amused with its light-hearted approach and unpretentious cool.

67 Hackney Road
London E2 8ET
07905 325215
Open: 10.30 a.m. to 5.30 p.m.
Friday and Saturday.
www.mgoldstein.co.uk

THE LONDON VINTAGE FASHION, TEXTILES AND ACCESSORIES FAIR

With high ceilings and streams of natural light, marble walls and frescos, Hammersmith Town Hall is a fine example of Thirties architecture and provides the roof for over a hundred leading vintage fashion dealers who gather to share their stash every five to six weeks. Pieces range from 1800 to 1980, all competitively priced. Vintage tunes play to an audience of fashion designers, costumiers, trend-spotters and students and set the upbeat but low-key tone. Items are clean, pressed and in mostly superb condition. Offerings bear dates and descriptions, helping those on specific hunts. The best collection of tea dresses hangs beside a stall dedicated to Gaultier denim, Westwood bustiers, Moschino PVC, Hérve Léger bandage dresses and Thierry Mugler bits, studded and structured. Regular stands show silk scarves in every pattern, print and colour. There are vintage Vogue, Butterick and McCall patterns, healthy dose of lace, cotton nightwear, the odd kimono and enough costume jewellery to sink a ship. Spotted among the cramped rails, boxes, baskets, tables is an Eighties Antony Price fur-trimmed green velvet prom dress and an Alaïa patent leather trenchcoat. The focus here is famously on quality; pieces have been picked with a keenly trained eye, so dream finds are often only a rail away.

Hammersmith Town Hall,
King Street, Hammersmith,
London W6 9JU
Stall prices £10.00 from 8 a.m. to 10
a.m., £5.00 from 10 a.m. to 5 p.m.
www.pa-antiques.co.uk

CHARITY SHOPS ON FULHAM ROAD

The Fulham Road charity shops now seem to congregate between numbers 600ish to about 850. Some degree of chance is inevitably present when charity rummaging, though you can be pretty certain of the following: 609 to 611 is YMCA and always has a number of suits in seemingly new condition. You often find great boys' tweed blazers and Princess Anne style jackets, cropped, checked and with gold fastenings. Trinity Hospice at 785 is a little more grown up – sensible heels and tailored dresses from recognised brands (they also have an eBay shop). Geranium Shop for the Blind at 817 is a fraction smarter in appearance and organisation; they cram structured bags into the window and house a selection of furniture (good for a mirror!). Fara, 841, has hanger after hanger of lightly worn designer denim and sometimes some rather smart bits for the home.

YMCA: 609–611 Fulham Road,
Fulham, London SW6 5UA
020 8616 0205
Trinity Hospice: 785 Fulham Road,
Fulham, London SW6 5HD
020 7736 8211
Geranium Shop for the Blind:
817 Fulham Road, Fulham,
London SW6 5HG
020 7610 6986
FARA: 841 Fulham Road, Fulham,
London SW6 5HQ
020 7371 0141

CORNWALL FARMERS

Provides great value for everyday necessities for gardeners, equestrians and smallholders. However, between the shelves of sheep dip and awfully practical commodities such as vast vats of Iams and industrial size Ecover washing up liquid (for not far off wholesale prices) one can regularly rely on shelves of classic Hunter wellies, traditional green or navy mostly, but on occasion they'll be a smattering of pink and purple. Chelsea boots, black or brown, zip up or pull on. Thrifty rubber riding boots scream of autumn/winter catwalks. Rather a lot of those great thick wool, ribbed sweaters with elbow patches and boyfriend Wrangler jeans!

Trenant Industrial Estate,
Wadebridge, Cornwall PL27 6HB
01208 812444

Open: 8 a.m. to 5 p.m.
Monday to Friday;
8.30 a.m. to 4 p.m. Saturday.
www.cornwallfarmers.co.uk

PETERSHAM
NURSERIES

Only a short bus ride from Richmond tube, Petersham Nurseries feels a million miles from London and closer to purest countryside. Near the River Thames and backed by Petersham Meadows you enter via a long dusty track. Petersham was saved and bought by the owners of Petersham House, Gael and Francesco Boglione. Its 150 foot herbaceous border and its kitchen garden supply the restaurant with salad leaves, edible flowers and herbs. (The garden is open to the public a few weekends a year.) The nurseries, teahouse and restaurant are to be found in and around a series of old-fashioned greenhouses. Furnished with elegantly worn garden antiques and original artefacts, which are for sale and carefully sourced from Britain, Europe, India and the Far East. Outside tables are covered with the season's best potted plants, many of which are grown on site. Pots, urns and galvanised troughs fight for space. In both the teahouse and the restaurant (for which booking is essential) tables are laid on the muddy floors so staff serve in wellingtons. The teahouse has metal seating beneath vines and a fountain view, while the restaurant, which seems straight from the pages of a fairy tale, has mismatched wooden furniture dressed with fresh cut flowers in jam jars. It's almost overgrown with lush tropical planting to a backdrop of venetian blinds and fairy lights. Food here is designed by Skye Gyngell who takes seasonal very seriously. The food is pretty as a picture but so simple that every ingredient sings clearly and satisfies completely. The restaurant leads to the shop, where alongside Skye's books are useful beautiful tools, seeds, garden twine, various vessels for flowers, Ilse Jacobson lace-up wellies, short or long for the lady or gentleman gardener, Fair Trade bathroom products and swish scented candles. Perfect Petersham is a magical oasis and giddyingly inspiring.

Church Lane, off Petersham Road,
Richmond, Surrey TW10 7AG
020 8940 5230
The nurseries are open:
9 a.m. to 5 p.m.
Monday to Saturday;
11 a.m. to 5 p.m. Sunday.
The teahouse is open: 10 a.m. to 4.30 p.m.
Tuesday to Saturday;

11 a.m. to 4.30 p.m. Sunday.
Petersham Nurseries restaurant is
open for lunch only:
12 noon to 2.30 p.m.
Wednesday to Sunday.
www.petershamnurseries.com

RELLIK

Famously adored and celebrity en-
dorsed, Rellik is frequented heavily by
designers and stylists who use it as a reliable source for inspiration. At the
dirty end of Golborne Road when you
think you may have gone too far, keep
going and you will see it beckoning you
from the foot of Trellick Tower. Co-
owners Fiona Stuart, Claire Stansfield
and Steven Philips met while working
on their respective Portobello stalls and
fused their creative visions into Rellik
and together present 'affinity, laissez-
faire, identity'. They specialise in different eras and designers, so customers
get the most intelligent edit. It is quite
simply where you will fall in love with
vintage; somehow it perfectly marries
the slightly chaotic with the considered in presentation. Arranged by labels for an easy browse; colours draw
your eye upon entry as rails of clothes
reflect from the distorted mirrored
walls. The best possible shopping scenario is to be somewhat specific with

what you might be looking for and
even better, ring beforehand; this way
the right pieces by the right owner
will be pointed out and you may be
guided downstairs to where the 'special pieces' are secretly stored. Rellik
name-drops everyone you want but
it's Steven's Westwood, Galliano and
Eighties English designer pieces that
are the most revered.

8 Golborne Road, Notting Hill,
London W10 5NW
020 8962 0089
Open: 10 a.m. to 6 p.m.
Tuesday to Saturday.
www.relliklondon.co.uk

BLACKMAN'S SHOES

The little and anarchic Blackman's
Shoes, run by father and son, opened
in 1935 as a purveyor of cheap, quality shoes to the Jewish community
around Brick Lane. Shoes come
from factories at times when business
is slow and thus it still satisfies its
cheap quality mission. They were the
first in the UK to stock Dr Martens
and today they are the least expensive
I've seen. Blackman's has a loyal,
mostly local fan base, for whom they
churn out £5 plimsolls in every

colour to complete the East London uniform. Furthermore, deck shoes, desert and monkey boots all come in at under twenty quid. Take cash!

44 Cheshire Street
London E2 6EH
07850 883505
Open:
12 noon to 5.30 p.m. Monday;
11.30 a.m. to 5.30 p.m.
Tuesday to Saturday;
8 a.m. to 2 p.m. Sunday.

ABSOLUTE VINTAGE

Absolute Vintage sells Thirties to Eighties clothes but one goes for the shoes. Heralded by *Vogue* as having the largest selection of vintage shoes in the UK (somebody said over 1,000 pairs at any one time), it certainly does appear that way. You can hardly see the walls and floor for all the pumps, heels, boots, brogues, sandals. The fairly recent renaissance (which doesn't appear to be dwindling any time soon) means the demand for Dr Martens has brought them here, worn and roughed up, in huge numbers. Everything is the very side of used but prices are reasonable for all but designer names.

15 Hanbury Street, Spitalfields,
London E1 6QR
020 7247 3883
Open: 11 a.m. to 7 p.m.
seven days a week.
www.absolutevintage.co.uk

THE EAST END THRIFT STORE

There is a certain thrill in wandering deep into the East End and down a still cobbled passage of anonymous warehouses. Among all this is The East End Thrift Store. Filled mostly with the later decades of vintage, there is a focus on the casual. Prices are thriftily low (I didn't see anything for more than £15) and you can join their Facebook page to learn of discounted boozy evenings. Endless rails of men's flannel check shirts, long and short dungarees, skirts and shorts (hemmed, rolled or fraying), and jackets and gilets. These are some of the better offerings. On site seamstresses are on hand to fix, hem or rework deliveries for a fast turnover.

Unit 1A Assembly Passage,
London E1 4UT
020 7423 9700
Open: 11 a.m. to 6 p.m.

Sunday to Wednesday;
11a.m. to 7 p.m.
Thursday to Saturday.
www.theeastendthriftstore.com

LABOUR AND WAIT

Country-kitchen-cum-garden-shed cum-artist's-studio-cum-beach-hut. Since 2000, Labour and Wait has been sourcing and selling covetable household utility goods from manufacturers who have stayed faithful to original designs. Stylishly simple, a lot has the feel of a Fifties kitchen with a big focus on enamel ware in dusty colours. A clothing range comprises pristine vintage work jackets, new but traditional artists' smocks, the best Breton tops and fisherman knits. Stock changes regularly but you can often find vintage buttons (complete sets), garden tools with a vintage aesthetic, rope props, plainest pencils and plenty of other accessories for the home.

18 Cheshire Street, London E2 6EH
020 7729 6253
Open: 11.00 a.m. to 5.00 p.m.
Wednesday, Friday,
1.00 p.m. to 5.00 p.m. Saturday;
10.00 a.m. to 5.00 p.m. Sunday.
www.labourandwait.co.uk

SILVERMANS

A leading supplier of kit to professionals of the military variety. Silvermans proudly supplies Her Majesty with footwear. It has a superb selection of boots and shoes; white naval brogues, old pattern but new leather nine-eyelet boots and patent officers' shoes are old favourites. It has some best quality selvedge and collectables from classic rucksacks to red Guards' tunics. It's with jackets that choice really shines at Silvermans: Swedish, German and US parkas with varying lengths and hood choices, very smart naval and bridge overcoats with gilded buttons, flying jackets (sheepskin or otherwise), MA1 in green nylon or black leather with or without fur collars. Prices are fair for what is undeniably the real thing in military attire.

2 Harford Street, Mile End,
London E1 4PS
020 7790 0900
Open: 9 a.m. to 5.30 p.m.
Monday to Friday;
10 a.m. to 1 p.m. Sunday.
www.silvermans.co.uk

KRISTIN BAYBARS

At number 7, where Gordon House Road meets Mansfield Road, find Kristin Baybars. 'This is not a toy shop', it says in the murky window of its cracked and faded façade. This statement soon appears to be plainly true; it is rather a highly specialist retailer for everything dolls' house, an entire world in miniature. Kristin's workshop/showroom/museum, rumour has it, displays 10,000 or more immaculately hand-crafted, almost bafflingly intricate objects by Baybars herself. There is no way to even begin to describe the variety that covers every shelf, surface and window ledge in chaotic, but narrative, scenarios. There is truly everything one can imagine – from more luxurious belongings one finds in the more opulent home – Victorian four-posters and dressers – through to everyday food and furnishings. This extraordinary shop, quietly eccentric, exhibits 40 years of slightly odd, possibly obsessive, art.

7 Mansfield Road, Belsize Park,
London NW3 2JD
020 7267 0934
Open: 11 a.m. to 6 p.m.
Tuesday to Saturday.

SABRE SALES

Asked when Sabre Sales began, Nick Hall replied, 'When I was seven, buying swords for 25p.' Hall's mother was then costume mistress for Southsea Shakespeare Actors, and Hall soon began to supply weapons for productions. Of course, when credited in the programme, no one knew 'Swords supplied by Nicolas Hall' referred to an eight-year-old boy. After years of collecting, a friend persuaded him to sign up to the police cadets. After promotion to the Bermuda Police he soon became very involved in designing, sourcing and displaying weaponry at Fort St Catherine. These displays remain unchanged today. In 1987 Nick returned to England and began to build Sabre Sales. Now comprising three shops, three flats and four floors of warehouse, it buys, supplies and sells militaria worldwide for theatre, film, fashion, re-enactment, murder mysteries, hornpipe dancing and strippers. Described as the tidiest shop in the business, customers are left to scour and build a pile of picks and then negotiate a price. Products are too broad to list but range extensively from furniture, props, saddlery, insignia and weapons, to uniforms, underwear, footwear and accessories.

The products are mint and after-battle distressed. Sabre Sales serves as evidence for the passion and knowledge of the fascinating Mr Hall.

85–87 Castle Road, Southsea,
Hampshire PO5 3AY
0239 2833394
www.sabresales.co.uk

BURLINGTON ARCADE

Britain's very first, and possibly most beautiful, shopping arcade opened in 1819. Beadles' liveried guards wearing Edwardian frock coats and gold-braided top hats (the smallest private police force in existence) did, and still do, patrol the Arcade and uphold regulations on behaviour. Originally there was to be no whistling, singing, playing of musical instruments, running, carrying of large parcels or opening of umbrellas and no babies' prams. The Beadles maintain the power to eject any visitor daring to contravene today. The Arcade has shops selling luggage, including the famous Globe-Trotter, clothing like cashmere and fur (to take you from country to ballroom), pens, sparkling antiques, jewellery with pearls a-plenty and intricately carved desirables. There are perfumes at Pen-

haligon's, where passers-by can sample the sweet scents from smelly bows in bowls outside the shop. There are watches, vintage and refurbished or perfect and new. Among these, there are many Rolexes in varying degrees of expense. Burlington Arcade is the definitive window shopping experience with smartly presented extravagant wares on show.

Mayfair, London W1
Open: 8 a.m. to 6.30 p.m.
Monday to Friday;
9 a.m. to 6.30 p.m. Saturday;
11 a.m. to 5 p.m. Sunday.
www.burlington-arcade.co.uk

WILLIAM GEE

Working with the Opera House and the likes of Vivienne Westwood is a surely impressive boast from the Dalston supplier of textile trimmings and haberdashery products. Zips are certainly the staple but they sell almost everything for the home or professional seamstress. They once thought of modernising but the customers protested; so it has remained relatively unchanged since its establishment in 1906. Floor to high ceilings with shelf after shelf of monotonous brown boxes house thousands of products. A long school-like service desk separates you from the goods so there is no browsing; a shopping list here is helpful. However, browsing and buying can be done online, although advice and personal service rely on a visit.

520–522 Kingsland Road,
Dalston, London E8 4AH
020 7254 2451
Open: 9 a.m. to 5.30 p.m.
Monday to Friday.
www.williamgee.co.uk

BROWN'S SHOE SHOP OF CURIOSITIES

L. H. Brown on Wilton Way, a former but abandoned shoe shop, is now inhabited by team LE GUN who publish the acclaimed annual periodical of the same name. A collective of Hackney-based artists, writers and designers, it fills the now named Shoe Shop of Curiosities with items as fantastical and bizarre as the illustrations in their yearly publication. Against a backdrop of brown floral and textured wallpaper and carpet in the same tones are artefacts, artwork and odd imaginings, punctuated with humorous junk: NHS-style glasses, almost

new Vans in textiles I've never seen (tapestry, velvet and cartoon printed), mismatched tea sets and glasses, and cameras I've never heard of, all to a soundtrack of scratchy vinyl.

61 Wilton Way, Hackney E8
Open: 12 noon to 6 p.m.
Saturday and Sunday;
other times by appointment.
www.legun.co.uk

THE LAST TUESDAY SOCIETY

A shop, hosting lectures and workshops by artists and intellectuals on their esoteric musings, and a gallery which fosters emerging and established artists. All aspects are curated by Chancellor Viktor Wynd and his Tribune Suzette Field and it is in essence a 'Pataphysical organisation' – a concept founded by William James at Harvard in the 1870s. The store sells and lends a terrifying display of objects: two-headed teddy bears, taxidermy, skulls and skeletons, to illustrate just a snapshot of this shop of horrors, which is the odder side of droll.

11 Mare Street, Hackney,
London E8 8RP

020 7998 3617
Open: 12 noon to 7 p.m.
Wednesday to Sunday.
www.thelasttuesdaysociety.org

282

English style from the nineteenth century to fairly up-to-date, 282's speciality seems to be leather. Boots, brogues, bags, Barbour, Burberry and biker jackets are in abundance. Most have a rather unisex theme, though tweed jackets come wide and manly, small, boyish and boxy or fitted and feminine. There are fashionable furs, heels and hunting boots too. Colours mimic those of the British countryside; all notes of brown, beige and green, but flashes of colour come from a spatter of Gina stilettos.

282 Portobello Road, Kensington,
London W10 5TE
020 8993 4162
Open: 12 noon to 5 p.m.
Tuesday to Sunday.

VIRGINIA ANTIQUES

Ex-actress Virginia Bates's shop has bejewelled accessories alongside velvet, chiffon and billowing gowns. The shop's fairy-tale interior is decorated with fabric, flocking, mirrors and memories; invitations, souvenirs and pictures from past couture shows and parties are framed in taxidermy domes. All is dimly but pleasingly lit with Virginia branded Tiffany lamps. Pieces range from the turn of the twentieth century to the Thirties. Despite the shop feeling brimful, collections are concise and very much themed for the English eccentric. This eponymous shop started in 1972 and few fashion magazines, models, stylists, designers or mere mortals survive without stockpiling from her rails.

98 Portland Road, Holland Park,
London W11 4LQ
020 7727 9908
Open: 11 a.m. to 6 p.m.
Monday to Friday;
by appointment only Saturday.
www.virginiaantiques.co.uk

TRINITY HOSPICE, KENSINGTON

Besides a lot of Eighties cast-offs in garish colours with large shoulder pads, best buys include worn but once luxury travelling trunks and classic Marc Jacobs pointy bow flats. Better still are brand new and packet fresh undergarments (from famed handmade heritage brand Sunspel) for £3 pounds or £5.

31 Kensington Church Street,
Kensington, London W8 4LL
020 73761098
Open: 10.30 a.m. to 6 p.m.
Monday to Friday;
11 a.m. to 5 p.m. Saturday.

OXFAM, CHELSEA

Bordering on boutique, Oxfam, Chelsea is well presented and pleasantly perfumed. The window alone gives tantalising clues to the donations this outlet can receive including white Chanel silk trousers and classic black Louboutins.

123a Shawfield Street,
Brompton, London SW3 4PL
020 7351 7979

SCHOOL UNIFORMS

John Lewis and Peter Jones tell pretty similar stories in their school uniform departments: own brand boys' cricket whites, shrunken school cardies (best in grey and maroon), sensible box-pleat skirts, grey flannel school shorts and scratchy box blazers. All items go from tiny primary school sizes up to 16 years. The oldest age should fit UK size 12 because nothing is fitted. Unexpected highlights are fifty quid wax jackets in navy and forest green, which surely give Barbour a run for their money.

www.johnlewis.com

It's very much a private school affair at Harrods and each institution, in their respective trademark colours, offers some delightfully English wardrobe staples. Claires Court Ridgeway has an old college-like colour combination of green, grey and yellow and the stripes adorn a great statement blazer, school tie and senior scarf. It doesn't get much more Mary Quant than a rust corduroy mini tunic from Hill House, layered over opaques. Nothing could be sweeter than a Garden House nautically striped pinafore. The same can be said of a Parkgate House spotty, round collar tea dress. Wetherby's tweed overcoat beautifully channels the Artful Dodger, and kilts from Claire Court College Maidenhead could be a 'beacon of tradition' or iconically rebellious when accessorised. There is no showroom so to speak of at the shop so find what you need online then when you visit you can be specific and see everything close up.

87–135 Brompton Road,
Knightsbridge, London
SW1X 7XL
020 7730 1234
Open: 10 a.m. to 8 p.m.
Monday to Saturday;
11.30 a.m. to 6 p.m. Sunday.
www.harrods.com

DESIGN ALSO

From her unruly premises in Highbury, Yvonne Lyddon has been an authority on bra fitting for over twenty years. You can hardly penetrate the shop for all the cardboard boxes gathering dust as far as the eye can see. Here the focus is not on the aesthetics, but more on function. Design Also is famous for fitting and finding you a bra but not so much for dazzling customer service or sumptuous surroundings. It stocks many underwear styles but you will have to be shown them as nothing much is on display. Rather bizarrely there is a selection of mother of the bride style hats and jazzy hosiery.

101 St Paul's Road, Highbury,
London N1 2NA

020 7354 0035
Open: 1 p.m. to 7 p.m.
Monday to Saturday;
2.30 p.m. to 7 p.m.
Wednesday;
12 noon to 7 p.m. Saturday.

CRUSAID

Loved by locals and supported by design houses and celebrities, Crusaid has an unusually party-like atmosphere; assistants are among the friendliest and the music is loud. This, along with generous donations (largely because of its exclusive postcode), has gained it its deservedly glowing reputation. There is a quiet library out back with records and books carefully catalogued into genre. A rail dedicated to Moschino is juxtaposed with formal men's dress shirts; there's often a Turnbull & Asser or two (great on girls). Good men's jackets and shoes are a given here.

19 Churton Street, London
SW1V 2LY
020 7233 8736
Open: 10 a.m. to 6 p.m.
Monday to Saturday;
11 a.m. to 3 p.m. Sunday.
www.crusaid.org.uk

THE HOUSE
OF BRUAR

As you drive up through the Highlands of Scotland and along the A9, you gaze upon the peaceful River Tay beneath the magnificent mountains of Perthshire. A scene like this leads naturally to fantasies of castle living and a fishing/shooting/riding moment. The House of Bruar rises from the landscape, a Harrods in Scotch mist, and satisfies all these dreams. Widely acknowledged as Scotland's most prestigious independent store and the home of the very best in craftsmanship, there is a focus on stylish country clothing and Scottish knitwear. The knitwear hall boasts the largest collection of cashmere in the UK; time-honoured classics do best like ladies' twinsets and grandpa-style V-neck cardigans. Most styles come in cashmere and merino. A close partnership with the widely stocked but unrivalled Johnstons of Elgin cashmere ensures prices are noticeably cheaper than any competition. Furthermore there is a generous selection of brushed cotton men's checked shirts made to Jermyn Street standards. Jackets go from quilted through hacking to shooting. Pussy-bow, piecrust and Liberty print blouses please ladies who want something more fitted than the men's checks. Hand-lasted traditional long boots, leather tassel loafers and everything in between make up footwear and there is every item you might imagine in the famous Harris Tweed. Other departments see equipment for all country pursuits: fishing, shooting, golf, boating and riding. There are also practical clothing and accessories for the discerning sportsman or woman. Pantry and homeware sections not only quench your thirst and fill your stomach but could fill your home with kit and bits for both inside and out.

By Blair Atholl, Perthshire,
Scotland, PH18 5TW
01796 483236
Open: summer and winter
opening hours vary.
www.houseofbruar.com

CAMDEN PASSAGE,
ISLINGTON

Camden Passage is tucked away on cobbled streets, just off Islington's main thoroughfare of Upper Street. Some permanent shops are open all week (often only by appointment) but main market and trading days are Wednesdays and Saturdays when stalls spill on to the streets and the atmosphere is at its liveliest. World famous for the range of shops, arcades, malls and markets on the Passage and the tinier roads adjacent, where specialist stuff is sold. There are antiques from all eras, jewellery, collectables, ceramics, glassware, lighting, furniture and silver. Saturdays, particularly, have some good clothing on show with more than a few good quality fake furs. A wonderful regular stocks remade and refurbished bronze etched stamps. Themes include nature, animals and typography and are dazzlingly detailed. These mini works of art range from £3 to £10.

Camden Passage, Islington,
London N1
Open: 9 a.m. to 5 p.m.
Monday to Saturday.
www.camdenpassageislington.co.uk

OLD SPITALFIELDS MARKET (THURSDAY)

The site of a busy market since 1638, stalls of varying themes operate most days. However, Thursday (antiques day) is best. There are sellers specialising in vintage clothing, some charmingly bedraggled cavalry jackets, and handsome old work shirts that particularly reference relevant trends. There is jewellery, furniture, decorative arts/objects and odd bits that you could only get away with selling in Spitalfields. A dashing young addition to the traders is Oliver Henry Burslem who has pieces fit for those achingly stylish classic furniture stores. He arranges everything with that sort of eye but sells for negotiable market prices. He has twentieth-century furniture and design, with an eclectic selection of styles: Art Deco, Danish, Vintage, Post-war British and anything that he thinks is good looking. Customers vary during the day – in the mornings you get a lot of the trade (interior designers, shop holders, upholsterers, furniture restorers and dealers).

Old Spitalfields Market,
Spitalfields, London E1 6BG
Open: 9 a.m. to 6 p.m.
Monday to Saturday.

ROWCROFT HOSPICE SHOP, TOTNES

Lovely Lynn, the manager of the Totnes Rowcroft shop (one of the largest in the Rowcroft group), says their donations are hugely varied and mostly come from the generous locals. In Lynn's three years she has seen everything from an antique piano (it took six of them to heave it down the street and into the shop) through to the kitchen sink (they have had more than a few). They have a retro day every September and a 'posh' shop upstairs for designery bits. They are about to introduce a £1 rail and run craft classes; the first will be all about customisation. Quality clothing meets bric-a-brac, though here it is sometimes more antique or specialist in nature. A friend nabbed a very good vintage manual camera with a charity shop price tag.

62 High Street, Totnes,
Devon, TQ9 5SQ
01803 863245

JAMES SMITH & SONS

If a business is still going strong after 180 years, it must be doing something right. James Smith & Sons is, even now, run by the direct descendants of the original Mr Smith. The business has always thrived, perhaps due to the English weather, but also as a consequence of the outstanding reputation the company has deservedly earned for their umbrellas and repair service. It is generally recognised that London is the home of the best umbrellas and walking sticks, and James Smith & Sons is thrilled to be able to continue that tradition. Still as it was in 1857 when it moved from Fouberts Place, this family business makes umbrellas, sticks and canes for ladies and gentlemen from their historic and beautiful shop on New Oxford Street, a stunning reminder of the Victorian period, retaining its original fittings. Brollies come with tassels, plain, striped, checked, animal printed and in so many other variations besides. Handles are offered in metal, glass, carved wood, fur, leather, bamboo and bone. The same sort of choice can be found for walking sticks. Made-to-measure type services are available from the suitably smart staff, who maintain a formal disposition.

53 New Oxford Street,
London WC1A 1BL
020 7836 4731
Open: 9.30 a.m. to 5.15 p.m.
Monday to Friday;
10 a.m. to 5.15 p.m. Saturday.
www.james-smith.co.uk

AIVLY

Aivly tack shop and country store is just that, but gone posh. It ticks all the boxes: feed and bedding, check; saddles, bridles and reins, check; rugs, stirrups and leathers, check; plus some specialist bits and a sizeable range of actual bits too. However, besides all this there is a range of boots that is beaten only by online stores. The best in the business is here and includes Ariat lace-up boots. Other highlights include smart Pikeur tailcoats and tremendously feminine Caldene show jackets with little fox buttons.

Crow Lane, Ringwood,
Hampshire BH24 3EA
01425 472341
Open: 9 a.m. to 5.30 p.m.
Monday to Friday;
9 a.m. to 5 p.m. Saturday;
10 a.m. to 4 p.m. Sunday.
www.aivly.com

SNOOPERS PARADISE

Snoopers Paradise has been a stalwart of Brighton retail for rather a long time. I have heard it compared to an American flea market. Indeed, it is Brighton's biggest second-hand shop. A village of traders, stalls and products are haphazardly thrown together. This most renowned market has over ninety stands presenting an almost overwhelmingly broad variety of antiques, collectables, jewellery, vintage clothing, furniture, old toys, retro bits and miscellaneous bric-a-brac. With this much choice it is easily Brighton's best prop shop. The majority of the lots are themed but you will still need some stamina. Unfortunately, there is no bartering here; all the payments are dealt with at a centralised desk but the result is smooth, easy purchasing. Its cult status in Brighton makes it a landmark and so prices aren't rock bottom, but there are still bargains to be had. There is some ludicrously ugly stuff but nevertheless there is no doubt that you will leave with a smile.

7–8 Kensington Gardens,
Brighton, East Sussex BN1 4AL
01273 602558
Open: 10 a.m. to 6 p.m. Monday to
Saturday; 11 a.m. to 4 p.m. Sunday.

SAVVY ROW

Savvy Row is vintage British classics, guaranteed. Paul Tiernan fell into the vintage clothes trade in 2004, when his father's rails of Fifties and Sixties suits and coats (too good to throw out) had no place when he and his wife downsized. Paul sold them on eBay but the quality, the detailing and all the history became so appealing that he began to actively source pieces to sell. His phrase for the classics he has chosen to dedicate himself to is 'permanent fashion' and this refers to Savile Row bespoke pieces, Crombie overcoats, classic tweeds, vintage Aquascutum and Burberry. 'Personality-wise the business is quintessentially British and mildly eccentric.' Paul gave up his day job in 2006 (retail manager for Great North Eastern Railway) and now employs three others at the County Durham headquarters. This online store makes things enormously easy: lots of images, clear and detailed descriptions, a fourteen-day returns policy and online and telephone ordering services. They say 'you can put together a classic wardrobe from the comfort of your Chesterfield club chair'. Future plans are to launch an own brand label, new pieces based on hard-to-find classic vintage.

0191 3737664
www.savvyrow.co.uk

OPERA OPERA

This is a British company, established in 1978. Optometrists, opticians and frame makers, Opera Opera specialises in the reproduction of vintage spectacles and manufacture of bespoke handmade eyeglass frames, spectacle frames and sunglasses at its very own English factory. It's a rarity these days to genuinely be able to stamp 'Made in England' on a finished product, but it can, and it does. More than this, Opera Opera is a major eyewear supplier to theatre, television and film production companies. Pincenez, monocles and lorgnettes tend to be hired but are also for sale. Just like the real thing it makes its vintage reproduction frames using genuine rivet hinges and trims, not mock pins or stuck on modern mass-produced sunken joints. Choose a frame from stock and select from hundreds of different styles based on designs from the Thirties to the Eighties; most come in four sizes and over twenty standard colours as well as tortoiseshell. Designs include NHS-inspired retro; others come adorned with doves or dolphins or swans. There are pilot sunglasses, a lot of bling and teeny antique glasses. There are heart-shaped, round or square frames as well as cat eye, avant-garde, surreal, John Lennonesque, Buddy Holly-like or

Johnny Depp-ish styles. When you select bespoke the company is thrilled to make a one-off copy of any vintage frame. It can be made from a photo or internet link. The result will be handcrafted and unique.

98 Long Acre, Covent Garden,
London WC2E 9NR
020 7836 9246
Open: 10.00 a.m. to 6.00 p.m.
Monday to Saturday
(after 5.00 p.m. by appointment only).
www.operaopera.net

ARTHUR BEALE

Absolute heaven for maritime enthusiasts, Arthur Beale established this ship chandler more than a hundred years ago. Saint James striped Breton T-shirts and the loveliest beanies by the same brand hang on show beside shackles and bolts of every variety. Ropes, buoys, bells and all the whistles one might need, this shop supplies any and every sea life essential, despite a far from ocean location on London's Shaftesbury Avenue. There is a workshop in the basement for manufacturing rigging. Arthur Beale is proudly specialist, employing the most knowledgeable of staff to advise on their nautical wares.

194 Shaftesbury Avenue, Covent
Garden, London WC2H 8JP
020 7836 9034
Open: 9 a.m. to 6 p.m.
Monday to Friday;
9.30 a.m. to 1 p.m. Saturday.

STEPHEN JONES

Stephen Jones burst on to London's colourful fashion landscape in the late Seventies. By day he was a student at Central St Martins; at night he uncompromisingly championed the style of the moment at the legendary Blitz nightclub. He would be exquisitely dressed, crowned by one of his own unmistakable creations. Contemporaries longed for just a little of his individuality and so, unsurprisingly, by 1980 his first millinery salon opened in London's Covent Garden. Those premises became a landmark for everyone from rock stars to royalty and Jones became an aid to their headlines. Today, in sometimes radical fabrics and with such compelling but diverse designs, he adds his touch to the finest fashion designers' shows. The retail boutique, design studio and workroom are still in Covent Garden. Distinguished white busts and heads in the deep windows recently displayed an almost patent black straw boater and a chic eye-print turban. The hats inside perch on branches, like birds poised for flight. His works are magical and wholly unrivalled.

36 Great Queen Street,
Covent Garden, London WC2B 5AA
020 7242 0770
Open: 11.00 a.m. to 6 p.m.
Tuesday, Wednesday and Friday;
11 a.m. to 7 p.m. Thursday.
www.stephenjonesmillinery.com

THE OLD CURIOSITY SHOP

The sixteenth-century Old Curiosity Shop was immortalised by Charles Dickens, and aesthetically Dickensian it surely is. Short, stout and dwarfed between typical modernised London blocks, the green and red façade is almost cartoonish with a precarious overhanging upper storey and a sloping roof. Inside it is characteristically crooked and cramped with uneven floorboards and and wooden beams; it is probably the oldest shop in Central London. Now an upmarket footwear boutique, it stocks a fairly bizarre range of own brand handmade shoes but with more conventional styles through collaborations with Trickers and Blaak. Least odd are sweet and

sleek lace-ups with ribbons for laces and horsehair winkle-pickers. They do sell a few other brands with a focus on variations of the old-fashioned brogue and boot theme.

13/14 Portsmouth Street,
Holborn, London WC2A 2ES
020 7405 9891
Open: 10.30 a.m. to 7 p.m.
Monday to Saturday.
www.curiosityuk.com

THE BRITISH BOOT COMPANY

The British Boot Company began life in 1851, both making and selling hobnail work boots. Skip forward to 1958 and the shop became the very first retailer for hobnail boots, and therefore an original shop. Very soon the shop became a one-stop spot for Skinheads and Punks from all over the world. By the late Seventies the shop had a new claim to fame through their close alliance with the band Madness, who not only religiously shopped there but featured it in several videos. The Sex Pistols, The Buzzcocks and others quickly became very regular customers too. Beyond Dr Martens the shop is also the main stockist for Grinders, Solovair, George Cox brothel creepers and Gladiators, and so can and did confidently declare: 'If we haven't got it, it doesn't exist ...'

5 Kentish Town Road,
Camden Town, London NW1 8NH
020 7485 8505
Open: 10 a.m. to 7 p.m.
seven days a week.
www.britboot.co.uk

THE CAMBRIDGE SATCHEL COMPANY

Satchels have been adopted, in relatively recent times, by students, vintage lovers, the fashion and creative crowd. In little over a year, The Cambridge Satchel Company is proudly accessorising many of them. The smallest satchel is ideal, handy handbag size at eleven inches; the thirteen-inch gives more room for your sandwiches; the fourteen-inch is A4 ready and the fifteen-inch fits a laptop like a glove. Batchels (rucksack satchels) come fifteen inches wide only and the music bag is the same scenario at fourteen inches. In all styles and colours (there are most of the shades you might desire and the choice is increasing), the satchels have the

option of embossing to add that one of a kind *je ne sais quoi.*

01223 833050
www.cambridgesatchel.co.uk

QUAY ANTIQUES

The widely reputed Quay Antiques Centre has seventy dealers occupying 9,000 square feet, over three floors. Goods for sale include large selections of furniture satisfying Georgian, Victorian, Edwardian and twentieth-century tastes and, of course, there are decorative objects for the home in these varying styles. The stock includes: clocks; period to contemporary lighting; silverware; cutlery; personal accessories; jewellery from period through modern to designer; late nineteenth and twentieth-century oil paintings and watercolours; vintage textiles and clothing from the 1860s to the 1980s (shoes and handbags too); Victorian and twentieth-century household linen and sewing notions; decorative and usable enamelware, baskets and other assorted kitchenalia; postcards, books and posters; a large selection of advertising material; and antique, collectable and quality woodworking tools such as planes, saws and chisels. They provide a 'Finder' service too.

Topsham, Exeter, Devon
EX3 0JA
01392 874006
Open: 10 a.m. to 5 p.m.
seven days a week.
www.quayantiques.com

F. NORRIS & SONS

Drive through picturesque Beaulieu, complete with village shop selling jars of boiled sweets, and you will find Palace Lane, and F. Norris & Sons, master saddlers, feed and dressage merchants. Founded in 1876 as a black harness and boot maker, the original shop in the high street is still in existence today. Persian rugs carpet the floors of this swish equine superstore. Bridles and head collars come plain in pungent leather and fur or bling adorned. Highlights for sure are Dublin hacking and competition jackets with velvet lapels. Kids' sizes are plenty big enough and their fit makes them suitable for less horsey wear. Pick Pikeur from the rail, from jodhpurs to Japanese-style collar shirts. The dressage section does everything from stocks to cravats, pins and Codeba Derby club riding top hats.

Palace Lane, Beaulieu,
Hampshire SO42 7YG
01590 612215
Open: 8 a.m. to 5.30 p.m.
seven days a week.
www.norrisofbeaulieu.co.uk

SMART TURNOUT

Stripes take centre stage at Smart Turnout, which until recently was hardly heard of outside the Oxford, Ampleforth, Royal Artillery and similar circles. The specialist label turns celebrated colours into hand-crafted essentials. What's changed are not the products (for most items have had over 300 years of being worn in the above institutions) but it is now a necessary outlet for the modern gentleman. The timeless pieces present the best of British style: 'vibrant colours, bold patterns and exacting craftsmanship'. What started for Philip Turner, a member of the Scots Guards, as just wanting the perfect jumper displaying a unique set of racing colours for an event at Sandown, soon escalated to favours for friends and, before long, took over when other regiments and Britain's historic schools and universities came knocking for knitwear in their respective colours. Best bits for

British birds are a handsome selection of university, old college and military scarves (like Sixties girls borrowed from their boyfriends), cricket caps (stripy like jockey caps), Royal Air Force striped pyjamas, old school and military braces in colours nicked from Eton to Royal Navy.

0845 129 2900
www.smartturnout.com

SEW DIRECT

The is the official and best UK site for McCalls, Butterick and Vogue dressmaking patterns. Find treasures in the Vintage Vogue department such as cropped jackets, swing coats and prom and cocktail dresses. For a modern approach, inventively highlighted by British *Vogue* last autumn, chose modern fabrics in period designs.

0844 880 1236
www.sewdirect.com

JODHPURS DIRECT

Ladies' and girls' cotton, cotton-nylon and nylon jodhpurs. (Nylon is the hardest wearing with great shape

retention for a highly flattering look.) They come unusually but beautifully plain with no garish branding. The fit is excellent. Choose from regular fit (which is rather high) or hipster fit. Choose the traditional, which models classic features including turn-ups and knee patches, or plain seat for a sleek look or contrast seat for a black bottom, back thigh, calf effect. Pick from shades of black, blue, burgundy, or canary, caramel, coral and more. Operating from Yorkshire as a family run retailer, products are manufactured in the UK and cater for all shapes and sizes including those lucky longer-legged ladies; prices are pretty pleasing to boot.

07958 290 297
www.jodhpursdirect.co.uk

MACHINE A

Previously Digitaria, this store/gallery (once a Fifties Soho tailor) proudly allows hotly tipped young names in fashion design to freely showcase their work through the shop but additionally through events, installations and exhibitions. Machine A remains infamous in the neighbourhood for its particularly controversial window displays. There is a mutual understanding between creative director and owner Stavros Karelis and his chosen designers. The concept is to establish these creatives without the aesthetic compromise of, say, being forced to be commercial. The mostly unaffordable pieces focus on an achingly contemporary and somewhat severe silhouette, but designs effectively flaunt these undoubtedly talented designers' skill and vision.

60 Berwick Street, Soho,
London W1F 8SU
020 7998 3385
www.machine-a.com

LIBERTY FABRICS

Arthur Liberty's intuitive vision led him around the world for inspiration. It is this spirit that has resulted in Liberty being synonymous with great design and luxury since 1875 and continues to thrive today in the iconic Tudor revival building constructed in 1924. A recent facelift has not only revived and re-energised the interior for its very modern clientele (while preserving the integrity of the beautiful historic building) but also places a bigger emphasis on the haberdashery department. In keeping with the surge of popularity in

craft and vintage prints, the design studio busily creates new and reworks classic prints every season. Themes range from geometric, abstract and animal to classics (flowers and foliage), fruit, leaves and paisley. Buy fabric by the metre for colourful, sometimes bold, sometimes even brave home furnishing or for feminine, striking, instantly recognisable dressmaking.

Great Marlborough Street,
London W1B 5AH
020 7734 1234
Open: 10 a.m. to 9 p.m.
Monday to Saturday;
12 noon to 6 p.m. Sunday.
www.liberty.co.uk

BADMINTON HORSE TRIALS

Badminton House is the family home of the eleventh Duke of Beaufort, the President of the Horse Trials; he was himself a very successful rider. The estate provides the grounds for the trials, an annual event usually scheduled over the May Day weekend. Watch dressage, jumping, cross-country and competitions, go on course walks and sample the catering. Picnic, then peruse, for Badminton is commonly thought to be the best show for horsey fashion.

020 7514 0016
Open: 10 a.m. to 6.30 p.m.
Monday to Saturday;
10 a.m. to 7.00 p.m. Thursday.
www.brownsfashion.com

BROWNS

Joan (affectionately known as Mrs B, of course) with Sidney (husband) created Browns in 1970. Once a small shop, just the ground floor at 27 South Molton Street, Browns quite rapidly became one of London's most important fashion destinations and kept growing. Today, the South Molton Street branch (one of a few) comprises five connecting townhouses. Credited with introducing us to John Galliano, Alexander McQueen, Hussein Chalayan and Commes des Garçons, Mrs B modestly claims this business of spotting future fashion superstars is 'nothing more than a hunch'. Big breaks have come for Christopher Kane, Mark Fast and Gareth Pugh relatively recently courtesy of Browns and there undoubtedly will be more, season after season. They edit tremendously to present an image of individuality but, just as importantly, an image of quality, too.

24–27 South Molton Street,
London W1K 5RD

CARLO MANZI

Over twenty or so years of acquiring, collecting and buying, Carlo has spread into three linked spaces plus one across the road. They are full to the brim. Clothing and costumes with a twentieth- and twenty-first-century theme are scrupulously archived, pressed and hung on rails, stacked neatly and repackaged on shelves or lined up and labelled in drawers. There does appear to be a slightly bigger nod towards menswear with suits as far as you can see. They range from everyday casual through to evening formal, every colour, every fabric and in every stage of worn. Apparel deemed too tatty by a vintage trader is 'gold dust' to Manzi. To boot, they have shoes and scarves, as well as coats, ties, watches, glasses and hats. Carlo Manzi rents out for film, TV, theatre and increasingly for designers and their research (they look at zips, buttons, flies and lapels, colours, cut, fabrics and stitching). The stock is not for the public or for sale. Whether clients have the most specific of briefs or need to be informed and guided, staff know the walls, rails, shelves, drawers and boxes intimately. On my visit private fittings were in progress; they were choosing for multiple movie scenes, costuming for *Carmen*, and Burberry had just left with a rail for research.

31–33 Liddell Road,
West Hampstead,
London NW6 2EW
020 7625 6391

FROCK ME!

Several times a year and now in two locations, Frock Me! serves both London and Brighton's vintage enthusiasts. Matthew Adams (qualified in costume design) was responsible for the first Vintage Fashion Fair, which was renamed as Frock Me! Preceding that, he had set up the still thriving Stables Market in Camden Lock. The top vintage dealers in the country come to Frock Me! to sell their unrivalled collections of everything you'd expect, and thereby sustain fans of the celebrity, stylist, model, fashion student variety. Periods from Twenties

flapper to Eighties retro are well served; additionally, those wishing to channel burlesque are certainly provided for. Prices range from single digit pounds to budget-busting hundreds. Step back and enjoy the pre-war tea room at the Chelsea fairs. A delightful room dressed with potted palms and antique screens, music tinkling on the gramophone. Cakes, cream teas and sandwiches, all served on antique china, of course.

Chelsea Town Hall, King's Road,
Chelsea, London SW3 5EE
The Corn Exchange, Church Street,
Brighton BN1 1UE
(beside the Pavilion)
www.frockmevintagefashion.com

WHAT THE BUTLER WORE

Lower Marsh feels rather far from the tower block jungle of Waterloo, but there it is, with its market and independents. At 131, What the Butler Wore screams with acid tones from the window and that theme doesn't dilute throughout. Unarguably the greatest variety of retro colour and print, chaotic and clashing but relatively ordered in its arrangement. It quite obviously specialises in the Sixties and Seventies, from all the mohair, maxis and minis to the shop girl's peroxide blonde mop. It's about being bright and blousy but feminine, flowery and fantastically fun too.

131 Lower Marsh, Waterloo,
London SE1
020 7261 1353
Open: 11 a.m. to 6 p.m.
Monday to Saturday.
www.whatthebutlerwore.co.uk

selection of 'great coats' referencing Withnail almost perfectly, though crumple and fray them yourself, as these come in near perfect condition. Owners Lee and Chrissie dream of extending to the basement for furniture and hire goods.

87 Lower Marsh, Waterloo,
London SE1 7AB
020 7928 0800
Open: 10 a.m. to 6 p.m.
Monday to Thursday and Saturday;
10 a.m. to 7 p.m. Friday.
www.radiodaysvintage.co.uk

RADIO DAYS

It's mostly Twenties to Sixties with an American kind of glamour. With that in mind, windows are strikingly sparkly. Inside and upfront it is like a dimly lit speakeasy and treasures twinkle from stairs and shelves. Such treasures include feminine fancies like vintage stockings, compacts, cigarette holders, perfume bottles. You can waste rather a long time rummaging through the old magazine collections, from *Playboy* to *Good Housekeeping* and everything in between. A clothing section out back is drenched in candy pink and among dance hall-ready gowns is a superb

CLOUD CUCKOO LAND

Rather typical of the Camden Passage vintage shop in its smallness and neatness, all drenched in charming. Cloud Cuckoo Land flags you down with ball gowns billowing in the breeze and it's as if you have arrived in some cobbled village, away from the city hordes (only a few façades away). You practically browse the vintage fabrics, patterns and feminine frocks falling from satin, padded and bowed hangers in private as you teeter on a varnished floor of old magazine tear-sheets. Fifties gingham dresses and net petticoats are particularly prevalent and there is an occasional designer name thrown in.

6 Charlton Place, Camden Passage,
Islington, London N1 8AJ
020 7354 3141
Open: 11 a.m. to 5.30 p.m.
Tuesday, Thursday and Friday;
9.30 a.m. to 5.30 p.m.
Wednesday and Saturday.

114 Upper Street, Islington,
London N1 1QN
020 7359 5284
Open: 10 a.m. to 5.30 p.m.
Monday and Tuesday;
10 a.m. to 7 p.m.
Wednesday, Thursday and Friday;
9 a.m. to 6 p.m. Saturday;
12 noon to 4 p.m. Sunday.

SECONDA MANO

The shop sign reads Giovanni but Seconda Mano squats in the basement of the Upper Street hair salon. On a fine day they might put a board out but have eyes wide open as it's ever so easy to miss. It sells secondhand but only just; only mint condition will be accepted. It is all about the high-end here and a balance of seasonal, vintage, classic and couture can be found within the comfortably chaotic closet-style store. The philosophy is as follows: you bring your unwanted bits along; they price them and mark the labels with your name; when they sell you get 50 per cent. It's rumoured stylists regularly offload samples and such, so you could perhaps spot a designer gem post-shoot.

UNICORN 50s DESIGNS

Specialising in quality reproductions of classic Fifties clothing, it has everything for any diehard enthusiast. Best is the range of Teddy Boy drapecoats in endless colour combinations. The shop itself is a dream in Fifties dress-up. Whether for fancy dress, or for a nostalgic moment back to the roots of rock and roll, Unicorn is it.

20–22, Avenue C,
Sneinton Market Square,
Nottingham NG1 1DW
0115 9110330
Open: 10 a.m.to 3 p.m.,
Wednesday to Friday;
10 a.m. to 2.30 p.m. Saturday.
www.unicorn-50s-designs.co.uk

359

PICTURE CREDITS

TRIBES

Plate 27 Two girls in riding outfits, Hyde Park, 1934, *Reg Speller/Fox Photos/ Getty Images*; **Plate 29** Punk girl, Essex, 1982, *Gavin Watson/PYMCA*; **Plate 31** 'Buffalo', *Reprinted by permission of Jamie Morgan and Mitzi Lorenz © (1985) Jamie Morgan*; **Plate 33** Dizzie Rascal, *Dean Chalkley/Ben Drury/XL Recordings*; **Plate 35** Teddy boy and girl, 1977, *Chris Steele-Perkins/Magnum Photos*; **Plate 37** New Romatics, *Caroline Greville-Morris/Redferns*; **Plate 39** Raincoats, 1979, *Janette Beckman/Redferns*; **Plate 40** Grunge, *David Sims*; **Plate 43** 'The Super Stars', Story of Pop magazine, *Land Lost Content/HIP/TopFoto.co.uk*; **Plate 45** Mods, *unknown*; **Plate 47** Margate, 1982 © *Derek Ridgers*; **Plate 49** Pauline Black, *unknown*; **Plate 50** 'Flash Lit Strop, the park', 1985 © *Tom Wood*; **Plate 53** Siouxsie Sioux, 1979, Ray Stevenson/Rex Features; **Plate 55** Emo, *David Sims*; **Plate 57** Nigella Lawson, *unknown*; **Plate 59** Cheap Date Swap Shop, *Kira Jolliffe and Bay Garnett*, from *The Cheap Date Guide to Style, Bantam Press, 2007*; **Plate 61** Rave, *David Sims*; **Plate 63** Nu-rave design by Carri Mundane, 2006, *Gareth Cattermole/Getty Images*; **Plate 65** The Horrors, 2007, *Titia Hahne/Redferns*.

TYPICAL ENGLISH GARB

Plate 66 Withnail & I, *The Cannon Group*; **Plate 67** Kurt Cobain, *David Sims*; **Plate 68** Adam Gear advert, *unknown*; **Plate 69** Ian Curtis, 1979, *Kevin Cummins/Getty Images*; **Plate 70** Vivienne Westwood and Malcolm McClaren, *Vivienne Westwood*; **Plate 71** Princess Anne, *Keystone/Getty Images*; **Plate 72** Patsy Kensit, 1987, *Brendan Beirne/Rex Features*; **Plate 73** The Barbour, *Kit Houghton*; **Plate 74** David Bowie, *Michael Ochs Archives/Stringer/Getty Images*; **Plate 75** School Blazer, *RealPD (www.realpd.co.uk)*; **Plate 76** Grey School Trousers, *David Sims*; **Plate 77** The Twinset, *www.vintagepurls.net*; **Plate 78** Morrissey, 1983, *Kevin Cummins/Getty Images*; **Plate 79** Film still from *Ratcatcher, Pathé Pictures/RGA*; **Plate 80** Bananarama, *unknown*; **Plate 81** Skinny Jeans, *David Sims*; **Plate 82** Oxford Bags, *unknown*; **Plate 83** 'On the

Buses', *Alan Messer/Rex Features*; **Plate 84** Phaze advert, *unknown*; **Plate 85** The Tour T-shirt, *unknown*; **Plate 86** Kilt, *David Sims*; **Plate 87** Jane Birkin, 1968, *Lipnitzki/Roger Viollet/Getty Images*; **Plate 88** Annabella Lwin, 1981, *Michael Grecco/Getty Images*; **Plate 89** Neil Kinnock, 1987, *SSPL/Getty Images*; **Plate 90** Grayson Perry, © *Grayson Perry – 'Claire at a transvestite weekend in Bournemouth, c. 1999'*; **Plate 91** Fantastic Mr Fox, © *Gerald Scarfe*; **Plate 92** Linda McCartney, © *MPL Communications Ltd*; **Plate 93** The Slits, © *Philippe Carly – www.newwavephotos.com*; **Plate 94** Lady Diana Spencer, 1980, *Central Press/Getty Images*; **Plate 95** Ian Botham, 1981, *Adrian Murrell/Allsport UK/ Getty Images*; **Plate 96** Damon Albarn, 1992, *Brian Rasic/Rex Features*; **Plate 97** Paul Simonon of The Clash, 1981, © *Lynn Goldsmith/Corbis*; **Plate 98** A giant print of photographer Polly Borland's work in Melbourne, 2008, *William West/AFP/Getty Images*; **Plate 99** Camilla Nickerson, © *Mark Lebon*; **Plate 100** Strawberry Switchblade, *teenangster.net*; **Plate 101** Film stills from *Mary Poppins* and *A Clockwork Orange, Everett Collection/Rex Features/Everett Collection/Rex Features*; **Plate 102** Alice Temple, *Richard Habberley*; **Plate 103** 'Self Portrait with Badges' by Peter Blake, © *Peter Blake. All rights reserved, DACS 2010*; **Plate 104** Elastica, © *Jeurgen Teller*; **Plate 105** Mr. Silly, *MR SILLY™ Copyright © THOIP (a Chorion Limited company). All rights reserved*; **Plate 106** Tony Wilson, circa 1990, *Kevin Cummins/Getty Images*; **Plate 107** Ringo Starr and Marc Bolan, 1972, *Estate Of Keith Morris/Redferns/Getty*; **Plate 108** 'Captain George K. H. Coussmaker', painting by Joshua Reynolds, 1782, © *2010. Image copyright The Metropolitan Museum of Art/Art Resource/Scala, Florence*; **Plate 109** Marianne Faithfull, 1973, *dietcokeandsympathy.blogspot.com*; **Plate 110** Siouxsie Sioux, © *Lynn Goldsmith/Corbis*; **Plate 111** Dunlop Green Flash, *Modern Horses*; **Plate 112** Wellies, *unknown*.

PINK

Plate 113 The Clash single cover, © 1978 *Sony Music Entertainment UK Ltd*.

TEXT PERMISSIONS

Page 48, quotation from *The Pump House Gang* by T. Wolfe, copyright © 1968 by Tom Wolfe, 1999, Random House, reproduced with permission of the author; Page 51, quotation from *Vita Sackville-West: Selected Writings* edited by M.A. Caws, Palgrave Macmillan Publishers, 2004, Copyright © Vita Sackville-West, 1918, reproduced with permission of Curtis Brown Group Ltd., London on behalf of the Estate of Vita Sackville-West; Page 67, quotation from V&A interview with J. Ormsby-Gore, V&A website (www.vam.ac.uk/collections/fashion/features/1960s/interviews/ormsbygore_interview/index.html), 2006, reproduced with permission of Jane Ormsby-Gore; Page 91, quotation from *Counting My Chickens and Other Home Thoughts* by The Duchess of Devonshire, 2001, Long Barn Books, Copyright © Duchess of Devonshire, reproduced with permission of the author c/o Rogers, Coleridge & White Ltd., 20 Powis Mews, London W11 1JN; Page 94, quotation from *Vivienne Westwood: A Retrospective* by C. Wilcox, V&A Publishing, 2004, reproduced with permission of V&A Publishing; Page 97, quotation from *The Fun Starts Here* by P. Yates, Bloomsbury Publishing, 1990, reproduced with permission of Bloomsbury Publishing; Page 103, quotation from *The Sixties in Queen*, edited by N. Coleridge and S. Quinn, Ebury, 1987, reproduced with permission of The National Magazine Company; Page 170, quotation from *Glam: An Eyewitness Account*, by M. Rock with foreword by D. Bowie, Omnibus Press, 2005, Copyright © Mick Rock and David Bowie, reproduced with permission of Omnibus Press; Page 219, quotation from *The Teds* by C. Steele-Perkins and R. Smith, Dewi Lewis Publishers, 2002, reproduced with permission of Dewi Lewis Publishers; Page 275, quotation from *This is England* by S. Meadows, Warp Films, 2006, Copyright © Shane Meadows, reproduced with permission of Shane Meadows and Warp Films; Page 284, quotation from *Jewels and Jewellery* by C. Phillips, V&A Publishing, 2008, reproduced with permission of V&A Publishing; Page 322, quotation from *Vivienne Westwood – An Unfashionable* Life by J. Mulvagh, HarperCollins Publishers, 1988, Copyright © Jane Mulvagh, 2003, reproduced with permission of Curtis Brown Group Ltd., London on behalf of Jane Mulvagh.

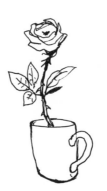